Walking

A Complete Guide to Walking for Fitness, Health and Weight Loss

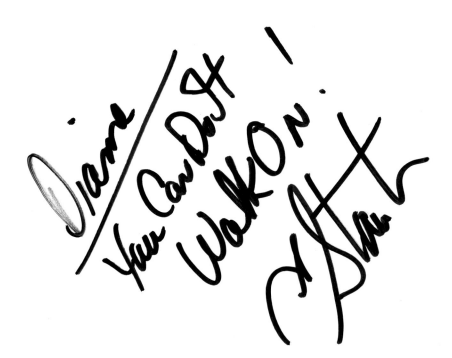

ALSO BY JOHN STANTON

Running Room's Book on Running
Running Room's Training Log
Runner's Personal Performance Record

Walking

A Complete Guide to Walking for Fitness, Health and Weight Loss

John Stanton
Founder of the Running Room

PENGUIN
CANADA

PENGUIN CANADA

Published by the Penguin Group

Penguin Group (Canada), 90 Eglinton Avenue East, Suite 700, Toronto, Ontario, Canada
M4P 2Y3 (a division of Pearson Canada Inc.)

Penguin Group (USA) Inc., 375 Hudson Street, New York, New York 10014, U.S.A.
Penguin Books Ltd, 80 Strand, London WC2R 0RL, England
Penguin Ireland, 25 St Stephen's Green, Dublin 2, Ireland (a division of Penguin Books Ltd)
Penguin Group (Australia), 250 Camberwell Road, Camberwell, Victoria 3124, Australia
(a division of Pearson Australia Group Pty Ltd)
Penguin Books India Pvt Ltd, 11 Community Centre, Panchsheel Park, New Delhi – 110 017, India
Penguin Group (NZ), 67 Apollo Drive, Rosedale, North Shore 0745, Auckland, New Zealand
(a division of Pearson New Zealand Ltd)
Penguin Books (South Africa) (Pty) Ltd, 24 Sturdee Avenue, Rosebank, Johannesburg 2196, South Africa

Penguin Books Ltd, Registered Offices: 80 Strand, London WC2R 0RL, England

First published 2009

1 2 3 4 5 6 7 8 9 10 (CR)

Copyeditor: Lee Craig
Graphic design: Nancy Gillis
Cover design: Nancy Gillis

Manufactured in the U.S.A.

ISBN: 978-0-14-317398-4

Library and Archives Canada Cataloguing in Publication data available upon request to the publisher.

Visit the Penguin Group (Canada) website at **www.penguin.ca**

Special and corporate bulk purchase rates available; please see **www.penguin.ca/corporatesales**
or call 1-800-810-3104, ext. 477 or 474

www.runningroom.com

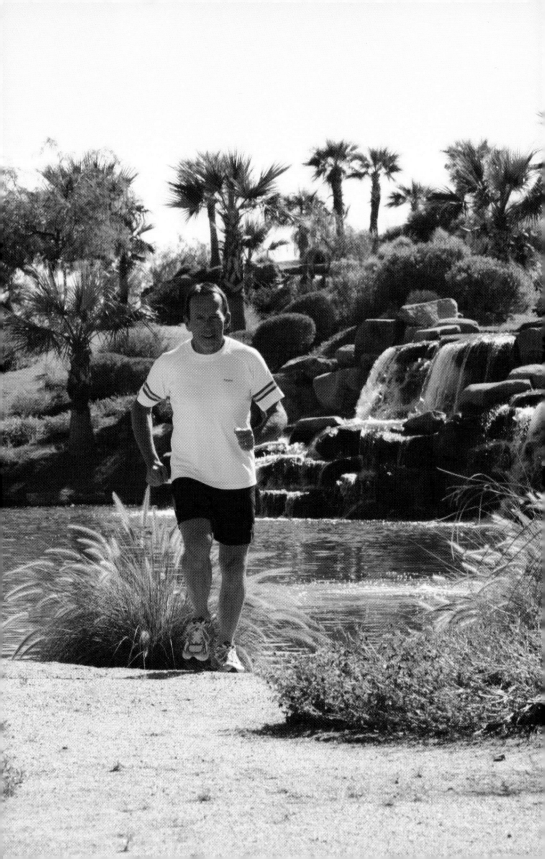

Contents

Walking and the Weather.. 140

Heart Rate Monitor Training............................. 152

Nutrition 172

Preface

Walking—the number one exercise in North America—is both social and personal. Walking is simple, yet it can be a life-altering experience. As a once overweight, two pack-a-day smoker, I know the power of exercise for personal change. The ultimate challenge is to commit to walking each day. You will receive a special joy along with a real sense of personal reflection when you make walking part of your day. Some days solitary walking provides you with both clarity of thinking and calmness, while on other days it is social. A walk can be just for you, the athlete, or it can be for competition, or maybe for completion. Group walking improves your health and wellness and at the same time expands your circle of friends. Solo walking works on your self-discipline and courage, whereas the group walks allow you to be like the child and think of your exercise as play.

Walking is an empowering combination of commitment and hard work leading to triumph, celebration and camaraderie.

Walking burns fat, rids you of stress, improves your self–esteem and helps you sleep better. Combined with a positive "I can do it" attitude, you soon find your improved sense of empowerment harnessing all your personal, professional and community goals. Each obstacle in your life transforms into a step towards your future success, thanks to a proven plan.

This book will provide you with an intelligent plan, one that is gentle, yet progressive in design. Within these pages you will find the motivation, inspiration, training schedules and innovative training techniques that will take you from walking for fitness to walking a personal best time in the marathon.

As a walker, you will enjoy the many physical, mental and emotional improvements walking will add to the quality of your life.

This book is dedicated to all walkers. Enjoy!

Introduction

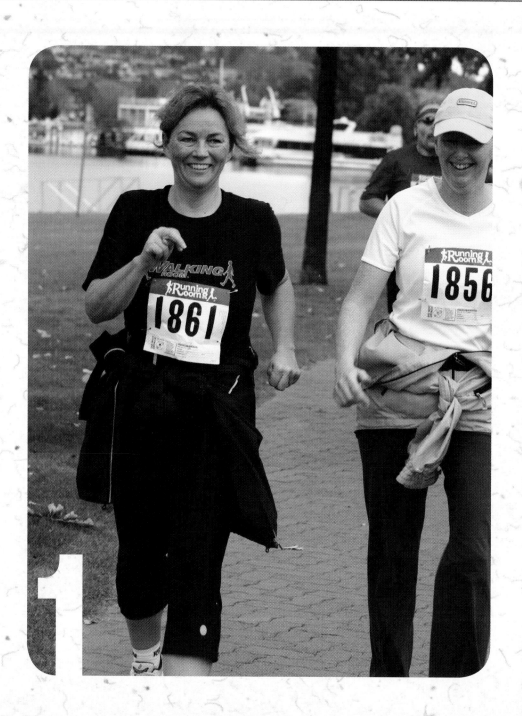

1

Using This Book

Walking—A Simple and Effective Exercise

1. Most people know that physical activity is good for them. Few know that physical activity does not have to be hard to improve their health. Walking is fun and challenging and helps you feel good about yourself.

2. You can design your own walking program by gradually increasing the frequency, time, intensity and distance you walk, or you can follow the programs provided in this book. There are a variety of programs, from the absolute beginner programs to fat burning and fitness walking programs to the distance programs for 5 km, 10 km, half marathon and full marathon training. If weight loss is your goal then you want to start at a very basic level and build up to 60 minutes of continuous walking five to seven days a week.

3. There are three program categories:
   + programs designed for people who are currently inactive
   + programs designed for people who are physically active on a regular basis
   + programs designed for people who have a fitness goal and may want to complete a certain distance and even complete a walking event

Benefits of Walking

After two to three weeks, regular walking will

+ increase your energy level and stamina
+ relieve stress and tension
+ improve your sleep

Over the long term, regular walking will

+ make you feel good about yourself
+ help you to achieve and maintain a healthy weight when combined with healthy eating
+ reduce the risk of developing heart disease, osteoporosis and certain cancers
+ strengthen bones and muscles
+ improve your self-confidence

Choosing a Walking Program

In this book you will find sample programs. Tell your doctors about your plans to start a walking program. Your starting point is to assess your physical condition and then choose a program that appears appropriate and comfortable. Once you have started, reassess your choice and if you feel you are overexerting, slow down. Alternatively, if you aren't feeling the effect from your walking program, try one of the more advanced programs, which will have you walking at a faster pace and a longer distance.

Assessing Your Physical Readiness

Fitness walking can be a strenuous physical activity. Seven questions from the Physical Readiness Questionnaire (Par-Q)* will help you assess your readiness to start training.

Questionnaire

1. Has your doctor ever said that you have a heart condition and that you should only do physical activity recommended by a doctor? Yes | No

2. Do you feel pain in your chest when you do physical activities? Yes | No

3. In the past month, have you had chest pain when not doing physical activities? Yes | No

4. Do you lose your balance because of dizziness or do you ever lose consciousness? Yes | No

5. Do you have a bone or joint problem that could be made worse by a change in your physical activity? Yes | No

6. Is your doctor currently prescribing drugs (for example, water pills) for your blood pressure or heart condition? Yes | No

7. Do you know of any other reason why you should not perform physical activities? Yes | No

If you answered yes to any of these questions, do not continue until you receive a doctor's clearance. If you answered no to every question, you may be reasonably sure it's safe to increase your physical activity.

*Questionnaire reprinted in part from the 1994 revised version of the Physical Activity Readiness Questionnaire (Par-Q and YOU) by special permission from the Canadian Society for Exercise Physiology, Inc. Copyright 1994, CSEP, Inc.

Assessing Your Walking Fitness

Are you unsure of your current fitness level? Where is your starting point? Just how healthy and fit are you? This self-test checks both your health history and your fitness habits.

Choose the number that best describes you in each of the 10 areas, and then add up your score. The results will tell you whether you have high, average or low cardiovascular health.

Cardiovascular Health

Which of these statements best describes your cardiovascular condition? This check is a critical step before you enter any vigorous activity. (Warning: If you have a history of cardiovascular disease, start the walking programs in this book only after receiving approval from your doctor and then only with close supervision by a fitness instructor.)

No history of heart or circulatory problems	3 ○
Past ailments have been treated successfully	2 ○
Such problems exist but no treatment required	1 ○
Under medical care for cardiovascular illness	0 ○

Injuries

Which of these statements best describes your current injuries? This is a test of your musculoskeletal readiness to start a walking program. (Warning: If your injury is temporary, wait until it is cured before starting the program. If it is chronic, adjust the program to fit your limitations.)

No current injury problems	3 ○
Some pain in activity but not limited by it	2 ○
Level of activity is limited by the injury	1 ○
Unable to do much strenuous training	0 ○

Illnesses

Which of these statements best describes your current illnesses? Certain temporary or chronic conditions will delay or disrupt your walking program. (See warning under "Injuries.")

No current illness problems	3 ○
Some problem in activity but not limited by it	2 ○
Level of activity is limited by illness	1 ○
Unable to do much strenuous training	0 ○

Age

Which of these age groups describes you? In general, the younger you are, the less time you have spent slipping out of shape.

Ages 19 and under	3 ○
Ages 20–29	2 ○
Ages 30–39	1 ○
Ages 40 and older	0 ○

Weight

Which of these figures describes how close you are to your own definition of ideal weight? Excess fat is a major mark of unfitness, but it's also possible to be significantly underweight.

Within 5 lb. of ideal weight	3 ○
6–10 lb. above or below ideal weight	2 ○
11–19 lb. above or below ideal weight	1 ○
20 lb. or more above or below ideal weight	0 ○

Resting Pulse Rate

Which of these figures describes your current pulse rate on waking up but before getting out of bed? A well-trained heart beats slower and more efficiently than one that's unfit.

Below 60 bpm	3 ○
60–69 bpm	2 ○
70–79 bpm	1 ○
80 bpm or more	0 ○

Smoking

Which of these statements best describes your smoking history and current habit (if any)? Smoking is the number one enemy of health and fitness.

Never a smoker	3 ○
Once a smoker but quit	2 ○
Occasional, light smoker now	1 ○
Regular, heavy smoker now	0 ○

Most Recent Walking

Which of these statements best describes your fitness walking in the last month? Fitness walking here means that you decided to walk for exercise, or chose to walk to a destination in preference to other means of transportation.

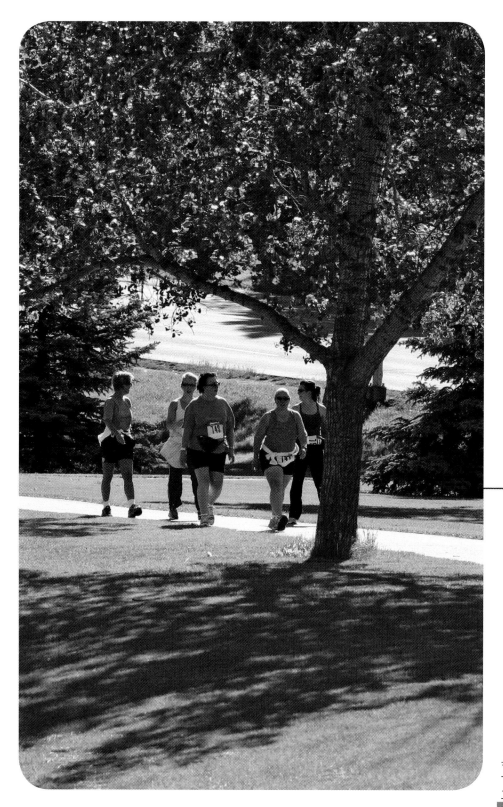

Walked nonstop for more than 2 miles	3 ○
Walked nonstop for 1–2 miles	2 ○
Walked nonstop for less than 1 mile	1 ○
No recent walk of any distance	0 ○

Background in Walking

Which of these statements best describes your history of walking? If you were previously active in these events, you will be able to use this background again.

Trained for walking within the past year	3 ○
Trained for walking 1–2 years ago	2 ○
Trained for walking more than 2 years ago	1 ○
Never trained formally for walking	0 ○

Related Activities

Which of these statements best describes your participation in other physical activity? The longer a typical activity session lasts in a related event (cycling, hiking, swimming, cross-country skiing), the greater the carry-over effect.

Regularly participate in continuous physical activity lasting 60 minutes or more	3 ○
Regularly participate in continuous physical activity lasting 30–60 minutes	2 ○
Regularly participate in other (non-continuous) physical activity	1 ○
Not regularly active in any physical activity	0 ○

Your Rating

If you scored 20 points or more

You rate high in health and fitness. You can probably handle a continuous walk of at least 20–30 minutes.

If you scored 10–19 points

Your score is average. You may need to take some short rest breaks in order to complete continuous walks of 30 minutes. These breaks are encouraged; they are part of your training!

If you scored under 10 points

Start gently. Walk briskly for 20 minutes, or until the effort becomes moderately uncomfortable. At this point, stop and note the time. Add two minutes per week to this time until you are able to complete 30 minutes at a comfortable pace.

Getting Started

Your fitness walking program is designed to cover three aspects of walking.

1. The Joy of Walking

For those who want to be fit for life, whether your goal is a healthier lifestyle overall or to hike around the mountains. The objective here is to introduce you to walking as a lifestyle alternative that will positively change the way you look at the rest of your life. Fitness through walking will become a part of your lifestyle and change your physical conditioning and mental outlook on life.

2. Athletic Walking

For those who love to pick up the intensity with some speed. You will become fit learning the techniques of power walking and of race walking.

3. Walking Back to Running

Walking helps many runners overcome inactivity or injuries.

Emphasis of Fitness Walking Program Training

Base training constitutes the largest and most important portion of every endurance program. For beginner walkers, there will be only two components of training emphasized in the first several months.

These will be the improvement of the heart, lungs and circulatory system and the skill, coordination and technique of walking.

The goal of this initial phase of training is for you to feel comfortable using walk and strolling combinations for 7 or 8 kilometers and for you to be able to walk 5 kilometers with an increased level of effort without significant discomfort.

Building the House

The Fitness Walking House

The training programs are organized into three levels, each with a specific role and characteristics based on three broad goals. Start at the bottom and build upwards to your goal. All of our training programs reflect the pace, intensity and effort at each level. Choose a program that fits you and your current level of fitness. This will change as you progress, so explore the various options.

Training Loads

You will find throughout this book that we frequently refer to the terms active, power and athletic walking. In addition, you will see the use of the term stroll in almost every program. The terms describe what we call training loads. These are terms describing the effort level and intensity of the various walking programs and training techniques associated with these programs. We will briefly introduce these terms here and go into more detail as we proceed into the detailed training programs.

1. Active Walking—Health walking
2. Power Walking—Fitness and strength
3. Athletic Walking—Speed or race walking
4. Stroll—Normal walking/recovery periods during training

1. Active Walking—Health Walking

This technique is used in our base training phase in our training program. This is the term used for normal walking done as a lifestyle choice. It is a term we use in our walking programs for normal walking. Active walking can be an introduction to increased fitness. It also gets you around. You are essentially walking for health. Most of your walks will be at your normal walking pace with little focus on time and pace. This category fits most people. It is the foundation of our programs, whether you are new to walking, want to lose weight or want to advance to our other walking programs. The goal at this stage is to keep a consistent pace and work on establishing a regular walking routine, building up to three to four times a week.

2. Power Walking—Fitness and Strength

This is the technique used in our strength and endurance phase in our training program. We use power walking to describe walking that is adapted to provide a more dynamic form of exercise than active walking. When you power walk, you are definitely looking for a workout. You are prepared to put some effort into the activity. Fitness increases through increased effort. You have a regular routine of walking three to four times a week and choose to slightly increase your pace and distance. The focus here is to improve strength and endurance through a brisker pace and longer walks.

3. Athletic Walking—Speed or Race Walking

This is the technique used in our skill and technique phase of our training program. We use the term athletic walking to describe walking that is faster—at a brisk to competitive pace; the focus is faster walking. These walks build fitness and prepare you for event goals. Fitness improves through increased speed and improved technique. Athletic walking incorporates activity to build your heart rate such as speed intervals, tempo and even race walking.

4. Stroll—Normal Walking/Recovery Period During Training

We encourage all walkers to take pace breaks, a period of gentle walking, used as a recovery from the brisk walk efforts. This stress followed by rest is the principle of all training programs. Think of rest as part of any good training program.

Phase I: Laying the Foundation

Your walk training starts here. You will progress through the three phases of building the house and achieve your ultimate goal.

During the base training phase, you get your cardiovascular system ready to handle future demands. You learn the skill of walking and establish a consistent program.

FOUNDATION

Base Training Phase
50% of your training period is spent in this phase

Active Walking—Building the foundation or base
Focus: Health walking
Results: Stay healthy and prepare for the next phase

Walks are at a relaxed to normal pace, designed to reduce your risk for chronic disease and an early death. As the stress-reducing walks become easier, add a couple of minutes to your walk every few days, until you're comfortable walking 30 minutes most days of the week. Thirty minutes per day is the recommendation for a healthier and longer life.

Benefits:
Substantial reduction in risk for heart disease, diabetes, high blood pressure, osteoporosis, obesity, clinical depression and a growing list of cancers. You will sleep better and feel better.

Focus on good tall posture. As you quicken your steps, expect your stride to naturally lengthen.

At this point you have a good foundation established at the base period. You have mastered good walking technique and have a consistent walking schedule in place. Here you will introduce increased pace and distance and may add hill workouts into your routine. Those training with specific event goals in mind will be adding hills and longer walks to strengthen key muscles in your legs and body.

Strength & Endurance Training Phase
30% of your training period is spent in this phase

Power Walking—Strength and endurance training
Focus: Longer walking
Results: Maintain or lose weight, gain strength and fitness and prepare for the next phase.

Walks are at a moderate to brisk pace; they are longer and sure to burn lots of calories and help you lose weight or maintain a significant weight loss. The goal is to maintain a moderate to brisk pace. Walk time increases to a point where you can walk 45–60 minutes several times a week. Power walking is a more dynamic form of exercise than active walking.

Benefits:
There is more effort, from which comes an added fitness benefit. There is a substantial reduction in risk for heart disease, diabetes, high blood pressure, osteoporosis, obesity, clinical depression, and a growing list of cancers. The longer the walks, the faster you'll lose weight and keep it off.

Focus on tall posture, quicker steps and bending the arms 90 degrees at the elbows to assure a quick, compact arm swing.

W
A
L
L
S

Base Training Phase
50% of your training period is spent in this phase
FOUNDATION

W A L L S

Skill & Technique Training Phase
20% of your training period is spent in this phase

Athletic Walking—Speed training
Focus: Faster walking
Results: Builds fitness and prepares you for your event goals

Walks are at a brisk or competitive pace. These faster walks not only build health and burn calories, but they boost your heart rate and tone muscles and build cardio-respiratory fitness.

Benefits:
As a fitness activity, the benefit comes from the effort needed to maintain speed. Substantial reduction in risk for heart disease, diabetes, high blood pressure, osteoporosis, obesity, clinical depression, and a growing list of cancers. The higher intensity provided the great overall cardio fitness stamina and energy.

Strength & Endurance Training Phase
30% of your training period is spent in this phase

Base Training Phase
50% of your training period is spent in this phase

FOUNDATION

Phase III: Nailing Down the Roof

You have proceeded through the base phase and developed your walking technique and established a consistent training base. You have moved through the second phase of strength and endurance training by adding faster and longer walks to your weekly routine. You are comfortable with the power walking pace and are ready to improve your skills of power walking and add in brisk and competitive pace walking. You do this by adding athletic walking sessions to your training program, such as interval training and even race walking technique.

Achieve Your Goals

Competitive Goals—Achieve your walking goals, participate in a walk with a specific goal in mind. It may be a time or distance based goal, such as 5 km, 10 km, half marathon or full marathon.

Fitness Goals—Lifelong commitment to health and fitness

Skill & Technique Training Phase
20% of your training period is spent in this phase

WALLS

Strength & Endurance Training Phase
30% of your training period is spent in this phase

Base Training Phase
50% of your training period is spent in this phase

FOUNDATION

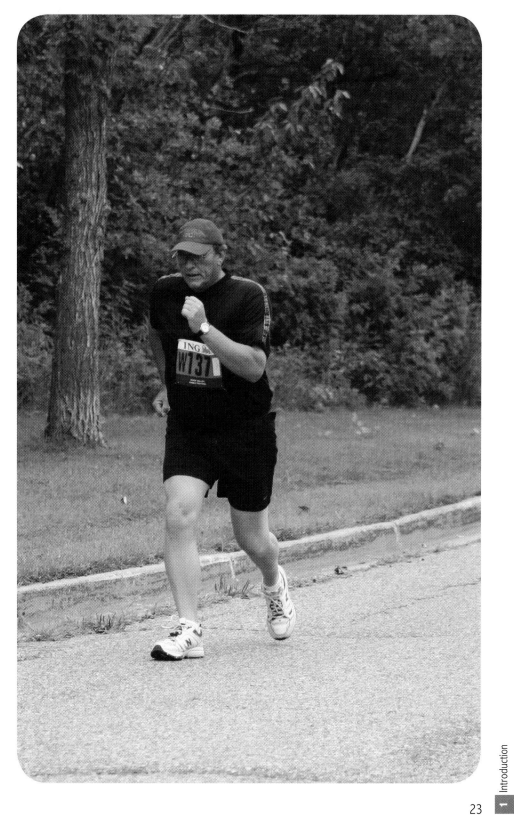

Why the 10 and 1's

The principle of athletic training calls for combinations of stress and rest to improve performance. Stressing our bodies at the same rate will eventually result in a slowdown with the buildup of fatigue, or worst yet, an injury.

In the weight room we do sets followed by rest in between each set. Track runners do high-intensity sprint intervals with light jogging to rest. Soccer players and hockey players call these sets wind sprints. Swimmers call them intervals. All athletes do sessions of high intensity followed by rest and recovery. Coaches know this more intelligent approach to training is a fast and safe way to obtain maximum results.

As we stress our bodies, we need a period of rest to allow for rejuvenation, where the athlete becomes stronger, fitter and faster.

Stress ourselves for too long a period of time at too high an intensity and we will experience a buildup of lactic acid in our bloodstream. This will result in that queasy, heavy-legged feeling. Our bodies are very well engineered. If we provide a short period of rest, it soon dissipates the lactic acid in our bloodstream and we feel fresh once again.

We know the importance of stretching; it keeps the muscles strong and flexible, which allows for better performance.

Brisk walking for 10 minutes, followed by one minute of strolling with an exaggerated stride length, is a way to incorporate stress and rest in our training. It provides a stretch to the muscles.

Stroll breaks of one minute during your walk training work from a performance standpoint. In addition, they remind us to keep up with our hydration and nutrition requirements.

Ten and 1's work; try them!

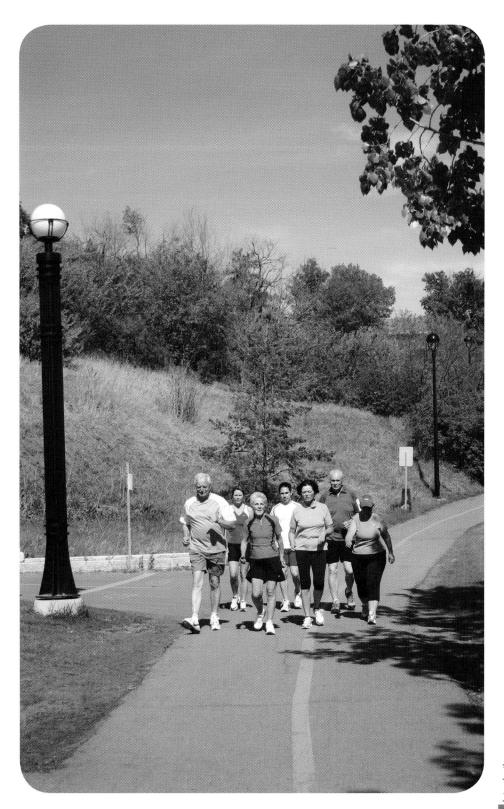

Smart Walking

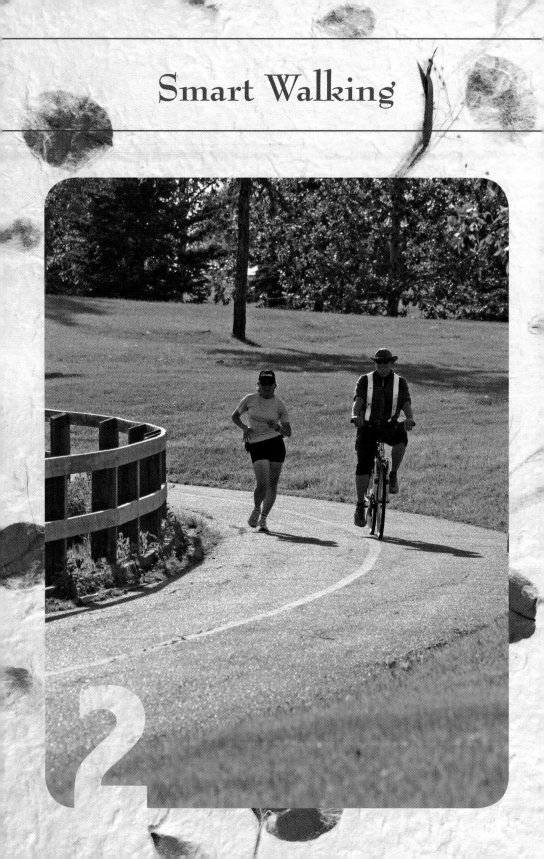

2

Smart Walking

There are a number of things we can do to make our walks safer.

* Carry identification. Carry your name and address, a friend or relative's telephone number and your blood type on the inside sole of your shoe or tied to a lace. Include other relevant medical information.
* Carry a cell phone.
* Don't wear excessive jewelry.
* Make sure your friends or relatives know your favorite walking routes. Leave the route written down somewhere. If possible, inform someone of which route you are walking.
* Walk in familiar areas and alter your route pattern. Know the location of telephones, businesses and stores on your route.
* Avoid unpopulated areas, deserted streets and overgrown trails. Especially avoid unlit areas at night. Walk clear of parked cars and bushes.
* Stay alert. The more you are aware, the less vulnerable you are.
* Don't wear headphones. Use your hearing to be aware of your surroundings.
* Ignore verbal harassment. Use discretion in acknowledging strangers.
* Look directly at others and be observant. Keep your distance and keep moving.
* Walk against traffic, so you can easily see approaching automobiles.
* Wear reflective material if you must walk before or after dark.
* Use your intuition about suspicious persons and areas.
* Call the police immediately if something happens to you or if you notice anything out of the ordinary during your walk.
* Carry a whistle or noisemaker.

Safety Considerations and Etiquette

On pathways stay to the right to allow faster walkers, runners and cyclists to pass. Avoid walking in packs spread across the entire path because it blocks the way for others and presents a safety issue as they attempt to pass.

If you train on a track and are a slower paced athlete, stay on the outside lanes. The inside lanes are normally used by runners and athletes concerned with time and the shortest distance.

Choosing Your Walking Location

Part of safety and smart planning is to make sure you have your walking plan made in advance. Letting others know of your location is an important safety measure, but doing so also helps you plan to get the most benefit from your workouts. Variety is the spice of life and so it is with walking locations. Mix it up a bit with a different venue throughout the week. It has the benefit of keeping the workouts interesting and also keeps you from monotony of the same workout in the same place every day. Changing the location of your workout also has the benefit of preventing injury. We tend to use the same muscle groups when sticking to the same location for every workout, resulting in increased risk of fatigue and overuse injury. When you change location you are also giving your body a break.

Trails

If you have access to a trail system this can add a lot of interest to your walk. Trails are generally compacted dirt or grass and are uneven in terrain. The softer surface is great on the feet lessening the impact issues related to the roads and sidewalks. The uneven surfaces can present some issues related to footing, rolling an ankle, etc., but in general the uneven surface allows your body to work different muscle groups as you work to stabilize your stride and improve your balance. However, trails can also be somewhat isolated, so for safety, always walk with a partner.

Parks

Most cities have great park systems that encourage walking and other activities. For the most part, they are well maintained and the asphalt walkways provide a stable surface. The advantage of most parks is that you can walk loops without having to go far from where you started. There is always a lot of activity in the parks; be aware of what's going on around you and share the path. Walk with a partner and avoid workouts in the dark.

City Streets/Sidewalks

Here is where you will see most walkers as well as runners and cyclists. Stepping out the door and hitting the streets is one of the benefits of walking for exercise and fitness. It's easy to do! You're generally walking on harder surfaces, so you are a little more open to repetitive impact injuries. A good pair of walking shoes will offset this risk. Be aware of what's going on around you. Streets are fast, noisy and crowded. Safety first!

Malls

Many enclosed malls have walking programs. Management supports the gathering of walkers who use the facility early in the morning. You have the advantage of a safe indoor environment. There's a whole social aspect to mall walking. It is a great option for a rainy or snowy day.

Tracks

The local school track or the track at an indoor fitness facility is a great location to walk. Tracks range from dirt, grass and rubberized surfaces. Having a measured surface makes it a lot easier to tell how far you have walked. They are also great for doing some of the more structured walking that we present throughout this book, such as tempo and speed walking. Remember, tracks are used by many different groups. Proper etiquette is expected when sharing the track.

Water Walking

Go down to your local pool and you will see that the pools generally have lanes available for water walking. These days many walkers use these lanes to work out without the impact of a hard surface. Water walking provides a high-quality workout with the buoyancy of water. The cooling effects aid in recovery. Further on in this book, I will provide some water walking workouts.

Treadmills

Many walkers have access to treadmills at the local gym or even have them at home. You can use the treadmill for any of the walking that we describe in our walking programs. They are safe and convenient and provide you with direct feedback on speed, pace and distance. They are a great alternative to going outside if the weather is bad and take away that excuse not to work out. On a treadmill you track your pace by kilometers per hour or miles per hour as opposed to minutes per kilometer or minutes per mile. One final note on treadmills: Most treadmills allow for incline, and we recommend that you set a minimum incline of 2%. This setting equates to the approximate amount of energy expended on wind resistance and changes in surface and elevation. The action of the treadmill aids in your walking. The perceived effort is less than if you were outdoors walking at the same pace.

Training Concepts & Terms

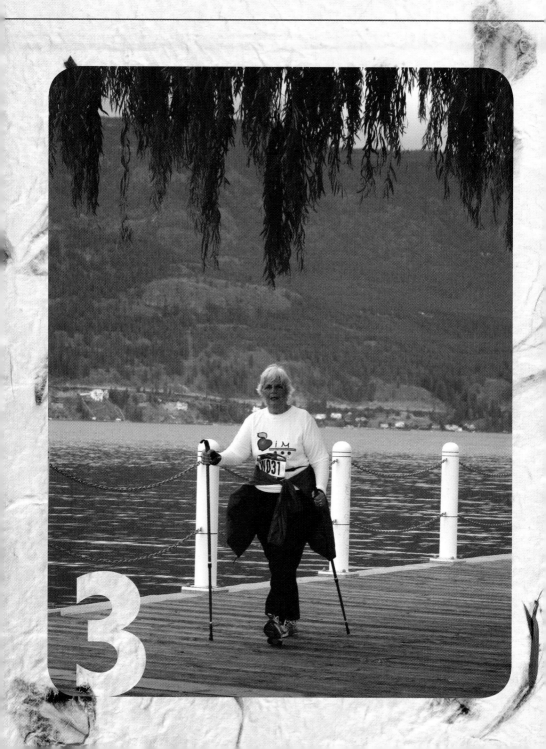

3

Introduction

The sport of walking and fitness uses basic concepts and terminology to describe what is happening with your body or why things are the way they are. It can be confusing, especially for anyone new to the sport. I will clarify many of the terms that you will see throughout this book and describe in detail some of the basic fundamental concepts that are the pillars of all sport training programs.

The Foundation of Training

Stress and Rest

Stress is another word that can be used for training. In brief amounts, exercise or training stress causes a temporary imbalance in the various body processes (muscular, cardiovascular). In response to this imbalance, the body will react by reestablishing equilibrium and will become stronger and more protected from further imbalance. This is called training. Over time, the amount of training stress must become progressively greater to establish an imbalance to promote further training.

Combine rest with training stress. Repair and adjustment to the imbalances of training stress can only happen when the body is resting. The rest period should be long enough to allow almost complete recovery from the training session but not so long that you lose the training adaptation. When the rest period is too short or the stress is too great, the body doesn't have time to repair and adjust —not resting sufficiently may cause fatigue or injury.

Implementing principles of stress and rest into your program will ensure an adequate training stimulus followed by an appropriate rest period. Even in the early stages of a fitness program, physiological balances can be reestablished in approximately 24 hours. Start out by exercising no more than every other day or a minimum of three times per week.

Practicing the principle of stress and rest will also ensure that the training stress is consistent. If a few days of training are missed, the body may lose some tone and endurance. A day or two of hard training will not make up for what was lost. In fact, it may hurt you in the end by causing undue fatigue or injury. The extra physical strain when trying to make up training will do more harm than just tiring you out, so consistency of training is critical for success. The individual who trains consistently will often see greater improvements than one who trains extremely hard at times and skips training at other times. Think of rest as part of every good training program.

Training Concepts & Terms

3

Consistency also has its rewards. As proper training continues, an individual will develop a solid fitness base. This level of fitness will ensure that when interruption to training does occur for a short time, loss of fitness will be minimal.

The stress and rest principle is the foundation of any training program. Its purpose is to ensure an appropriate training stress, an adequate rest period, and a consistent pattern of exercise to keep your walking fun!

The Components of Sports Training

Sports training has some basic components. All sports and physical activities have common physiological ingredients. They are mixed in greatly different proportions for different activities. The list below tells you a little about each. For our walking programs, we concentrate on these:

Endurance and stamina	Skill and coordination
Strength	Speed and power

Endurance/Stamina

Endurance must be developed first, because without it most other types of training cannot be repeated enough to develop the other components of fitness. In this program, building an endurance base is the primary emphasis. Building a base will train the cardiovascular system to better handle the demands of exercise and will train the specific muscles involved to go the distance. The heart will become stronger and more efficient at delivering oxygenated blood to the muscles. The muscles will become more efficient at using oxygen for energy and become more resistant to muscular fatigue. These training adaptations lead to improved aerobic fitness.

The most common way of developing aerobic fitness is with regular continuous aerobic exercise. Exercise of this nature should be intense enough to raise the heart rate to the 130–150 bpm range or 60–70% of your minimum current heart rate and should be maintained for at least 20–30 minutes. You should be able to talk comfortably while walking. So, do the walk/talk test! Muscular endurance is developed somewhat during continuous aerobic training. Weight training or cross training can sometimes be used to combine both muscular endurance and aerobic training.

This muscular endurance is also developed during continuous aerobic training, especially as your walks get longer.

Strength

All human motion is muscular. Stronger muscles deliver increased fitness to your walking or any desired activity.

Strength can be an aspect of general conditioning, or it can be targeted to specific activities. Strength programs can be designed for both speed and endurance. Strength can be improved regardless of your gender or age with only some restrictions on programs for young athletes.

Skill/Coordination

In sports walking, skill and coordination help you perform better. Skill and coordination are components of all activities to a greater or lesser degree. For walkers, your skill and coordination is increasingly important if you want to walk faster.

Speed/Power

Speed is critical to high-level performance. Endurance activity, like speed walking, comes from the higher levels of our endurance that keeps our muscles going under increasing fatigue.

The Emphasis of Fitness Walking Training

Base Training

Base training constitutes the largest and most important portion of every endurance program. For beginning walkers, there will be only two components of training emphasized in the first several months.

These components will be the improvement of the heart, lungs and circulatory system and the skill, coordination and technique of walking.

The goal of this initial phase of training is for you to feel comfortable doing 7 or 8 kilometers using walk and strolling combinations. You are able to walk 5 kilometers briskly without significant discomfort.

Hard Easy Principle

The body adjusts to exercise through adaptation, which is the enhancing of the systems of the body that were stressed by the exercise. Adaptation occurs when the body is resting from the stress of the exercise. Therefore both exercise and rest are necessary for improvement: Exercise and rest lead to adaptation and improved fitness.

Well-planned training systems respect this principle by alternating harder sessions with easier ones. The easier sessions may be days of complete rest or some other activity. A change of activity is known as cross-training. One day per week of full rest without training is common even among very advanced athletes.

The volume and the intensity of training are also increased gradually and with care. Increments of 10% have been found to provide an effective training load while avoiding excess training stress.

Excess stress does not allow adaptation to occur. It produces injury, overtraining and illness. Following training, the feeling should be one of pleasant tiredness resulting from a satisfying accomplishment. The accumulation of fatigue is a danger sign in athletes of all levels.

Walking Pace and Types

Race Walking

Walking pace is used in race events, from the 5K to the marathon distance. Many race directors now recognize walkers by age group divisions similar to runners' competitive categories. Runners have welcomed the addition of walkers to their running events.

Stroll Breaks

Stroll walks are used for pace breaks, which provide recovery between faster walking periods. They are always used in long walks or base building walks where it is important to develop aerobic endurance. We encourage all walkers to take stroll breaks. These periods of gentle walking are used to recover from the brisk walk periods.

Recovery Walks

One of the most important aspects of training is the recovery period between workouts. Don't always go at full intensity. This is why the recovery walk is part of the foundation of all walking programs. During the recovery period, the body rebuilds to resist workout stress. This rebuilding and adaptation is when the training effect occurs, which makes you stronger and better able to resist the stress.

You might assume that complete rest for some period between workouts might provide optimal rebuilding. However, it has been shown that low-level activity, especially that which simulates the activity being trained for, is better than total

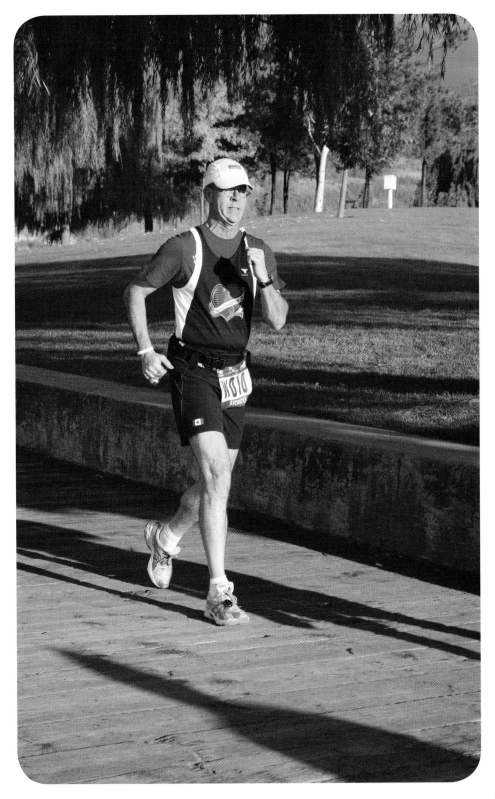

rest. It promotes circulation and stimulates growth of new tissue in a manner that aligns it with the activity.

Most walkers require 48 hours or more to recover from a hard, high intensity or long workout. Training plans often include alternate hard and easy walks in order to get a good combination of stress and recovery.

The purpose of a recovery walk is to recover from a high-intensity or long training walk and to stimulate circulation and adaptation to walking stresses. Think of these recovery walks as a massage to gently recover from the harder efforts.

Steady Walks Should Be at Low Intensity and of Short Distance

Intensity—Is less than 70% effort. This is a relaxed aerobic pace where you could easily carry on a conversation with someone.

Distance—Less than 10% of total weekly training mileage.

Long Walks

The long walk is a key element in aerobic endurance training. Long slow walks stimulate the use of all energy systems, including the use of muscle and blood glycogen with oxygen and burning fat. They promote the development of capillaries, mitochondria and oxidative enzymes that aid these energy systems. All of these changes benefit aerobic walking from 5K to a marathon. Long slow walks are a critical part of training for both. Without them, walkers do not develop sufficient energy sources to supply themselves for longer distance goals.

In addition to physiological benefits, there are significant psychological benefits in simulating the distance or duration of the event you are training for.

Long walks should be at low intensity (60–70% of your maximum heart rate). The object is to train for endurance, not speed.

A single long walk often comprises 30–40% of a walker's weekly mileage. Therefore, special care must be taken to assure adequate recovery. Doing so usually means two easy days of recovery or a reduced weekly workload following a long walk.

Strength Building Walks

Endurance training will often include strength building midweek. Do hills and tempo walking to build a strength base in Phase 2 of your training period. As in the long walk, they are intended to stimulate aerobic energy systems and build aerobic endurance.

Nutrition and Walking

Burning Calories

Weight is determined mostly by how many calories you burn compared to how many you eat each day. To lose weight, you need to increase your activity to burn more calories and you need to eat fewer calories each day.

A pound of fat equals 3500 calories. To lose one pound a week you need to expend 3500 more calories than you eat that week, whether through increased activity or decreased eating or both. Losing one to two pounds of fat a week is a sensible goal. You will want to use the combination of increased activity and eating less to total 3500 calories for seven days. Having intelligent and realistic goals will yield you the greatest results.

How to Burn Calories

Time does not matter as much as distance. If you walk a mile in 13 minutes or less, you will be burning more calories per mile. But for most beginner walkers, it is best to increase the distance before working on speed. A simple rule of thumb is 100 calories per mile for a 160-pound person.

Note About Calorie Burning:

You burn more calories per mile at very low speeds because you are basically stopping and starting with each step and your momentum isn't helping to carry you along. Meanwhile, at very high walking speeds you are using more muscle groups with your arm motion and your brisk walking stride. Using those extra muscles burns up extra calories with each step. Walking may burn more calories per mile because there is an up and down motion that lifts your weight off the ground as well as moving it forward.

The Best Way to Burn More Calories: Walk Farther

Build up in order to walk longer distances. Concentrate your training on building distance before you build speed, and walking five or six days a week. The calories burned by an extra few minutes of walking far overcome any other changes you can make.

Terms Referenced in Training Programs

Easy and Hard Workout Variety

You should alternate easy days with harder days. Easy and hard have these three variables:

Distance

A hard distance day is one of long, slow distances. This day is for mileage building. If you are training for a half marathon or marathon, you do this one day each week.

Speed

A hard day is one done with a fast workout, but at a shorter distance than your goal distance.

Strength

A hard day for strength would be one with hills or on a hilly trail. These walks work muscles you don't use on flat and/or smooth surface walks. They improve your balance. These are the same muscles used in sessions.

Base

This is really the sum total of all your regular daily walks, either long or short. The basic foundation of a training program is built around a base of good solid walks. Walking other than base training includes types such as speed, fartlek, etc.

Action

Base walking includes the total of the weekly long session and other moderate endurance sessions inclusive of those done on easier days.

Purpose

Base walking raises your metabolic rate and anaerobic threshold.

Long Walk

Action

The long walk is the longest session of your training program, building from 60–70% of maximum heart rate.

Purpose

The long walk builds muscular endurance by increasing the capillary network in the working muscles. It raises the anaerobic threshold, so that more training is possible in the aerobic zone.

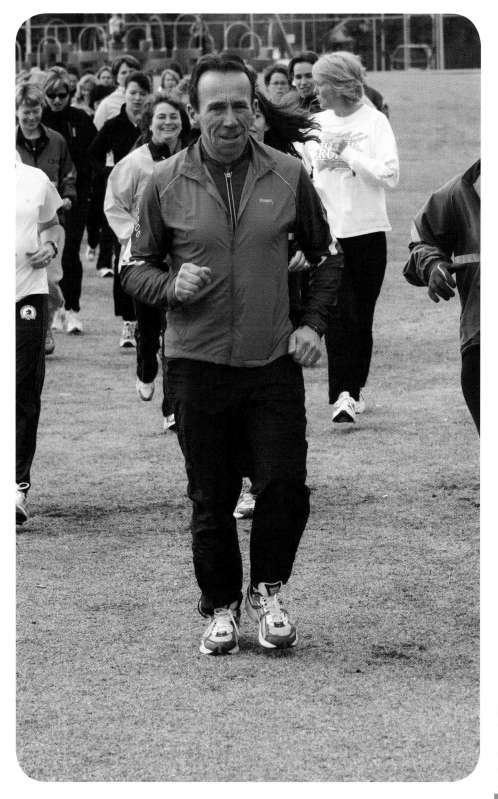

Tempo

Tempo walks are continuous walks at 80% of maximum heart rate for less than race distance. They can be either the entire session or part of a longer one.

Purpose

Tempo walks develop stamina and pace judgment.

Sample #1

Warm up for 10 minutes at an easy pace, followed by stretching and flexibility exercises.
Walk 20–30 minutes at 80% of your maximum heart rate.
You will be breathing very hard and able to speak only in short phrases.
Cool down with 10 minutes at an easy pace.

Sample #2

Warm up for 10 minutes at an easy walking pace.
Walk fast for eight minutes or 1 kilometer. Then slow down to an easy pace for two minutes.

Repeat three to four times.
Cool down for 10 minutes at an easy pace.
The threshold pace is strenuous, but one you could maintain throughout 10 kilometers. You will be breathing very hard and able to speak only in short phrases.

Hill Repeats

Action

Hills repeats are repeated efforts up and down a hill with a grade of no more than 10% (hard up the hill, easy down).

Purpose

Hill repeats develop muscular strength and raise the aerobic threshold.

Fartlek

Action

Fartleks are continuous sessions with a change of pace for various distances of the athlete's choosing. Do short bursts at 70–80% effort, and then have recovery periods to bring the heart rate down to 120 bpm.

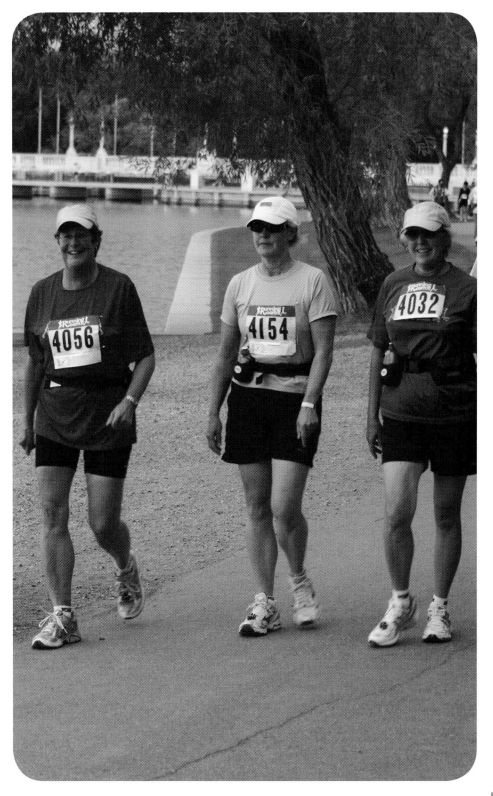

Fartleks build determination and strength. Fartleks teach a walker to walk at a varied tempo instead of locking in to one pace. Doing so will make a walker stronger over a course that has varying terrain. Fartleks can help a walker learn to stay with their competitors during a surge in the middle of a race.

Speed Intervals

Action

These are fast walks over short distances, usually with a relatively long period of recovery to allow the unpleasant side effects of the anaerobic activity to diminish. E.g., 6 X 200 meters.

Purpose

Speed intervals develop speed endurance, buffer the effects of anaerobic activity and improve coordination.

Interval Training

In the introductory and intermediate 10-week conditioning programs (Chapter 7) you will become familiar with the concept of interval training and its structure. But all we have done up to now is scratch the surface of its potential as a training vehicle by starting with some gentle repetitions and building into some speed play. In the advanced program, we look more closely at interval training. Here, we realize that we have at our disposal a training resource that is limited only by our imagination.

Interval training can be challenging! After some of your speed play, you probably ended up pleasantly tired, but elated.

As you enter the advanced program, you need to understand the principles behind interval training. As you progress, you find yourself constantly reviewing your training logs and the results of previous sessions. You use this information to move your present training to the next level.

Interval workouts are done in relative comfort. They have four elements: the length of the effort, the number of repetitions, speed and the amount of recovery time you take between each element.

Start from your basic workout. When the same amount of work can be done with less recovery than previously, you can increase the amount of repetitions that you do. When you've achieved that progression, you can increase the length of each repetition, further increasing the total distance you cover at a rhythm you can handle while maintaining your form.

The speed of the effort is the last thing to be increased. Don't attempt to increase your speed until you have achieved progress at the original pace.

There will be a natural improvement in speed as your muscles and your fitness respond to the training. Keep your personal rhythm and form steady even as you tire.

If you're able to do 8 x 200 meters in relative comfort, take 90 seconds to rest between each one.

Now build on this: Keeping everything else the same, reduce the recovery to 75 seconds. There will be a noticeable increase in effort.

As you progress, your total distance will increase significantly, and so will your training results. There will be some gains in speed as you increase your fitness. Repeat the sequence a second time, reducing the recovery to 60 seconds. Do another set with longer repetitions when you feel ready for the challenge.

Walking Sample Interval Sessions
Speed
These interval walking workouts increase your athletic performance by bringing your body up to the anaerobic threshold. These workouts are used by race walkers to improve their VO2 maximum (the highest amount of oxygen one can consume during exercise). It improves endurance and intensity.

Sample #1
Start at an easy pace for 5–10 minutes.
Continue, walking at a pace that brings your heart rate up to 80–90% of MHR for no more than 50 minutes. This is a fast pace where you are breathing very hard and can only speak in short phrases. End with five minutes of gentle stretching and flexibility exercises

Sample #2
Walk fast for eight minutes or 1 kilometer at 80–85% of your maximum heart rate. Then slow down to an easy pace for two minutes. Repeat three to four times.

Sample #3

First you warm up with an easy 5–10 minute walk, slow easy pace. Then the interval: Walk as fast as you can (gets the HR up) for 30 seconds, the equivalent of two city blocks. The goal here is to walk fast for 30 seconds, rest or stroll and then walk fast again for a 30 second interval. Each interval is approximately 200 meters in distance.

Once this is completed, you will do two minutes of fast-walking repeats 8–12 times with a rest or stroll between. Finish off with an easy 5 minutes cooldown of a slow easy walk.

Sample #4

Warm up for 10–20 minutes at an easy pace, stretch and do flexibility exercises.
Take off at a moderate pace for two minutes and then speed up to walk as fast as you can for 200 meters/yards.
Slow to a moderate pace for 200 meters (about two city blocks).
Speed up again for 200 meters as fast as you can.
Repeat 8–12 times.
Finish with 10–20 minutes of easy walking, followed by stretching.

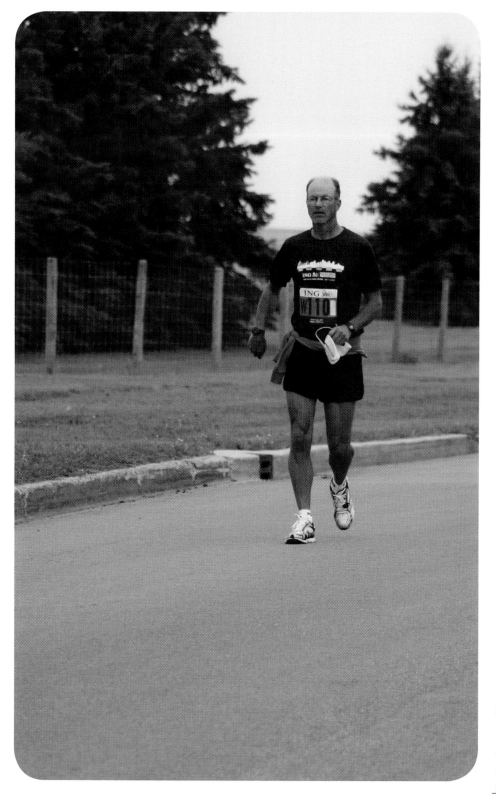

3 Training Concepts & Terms

Developing Your Walking Program

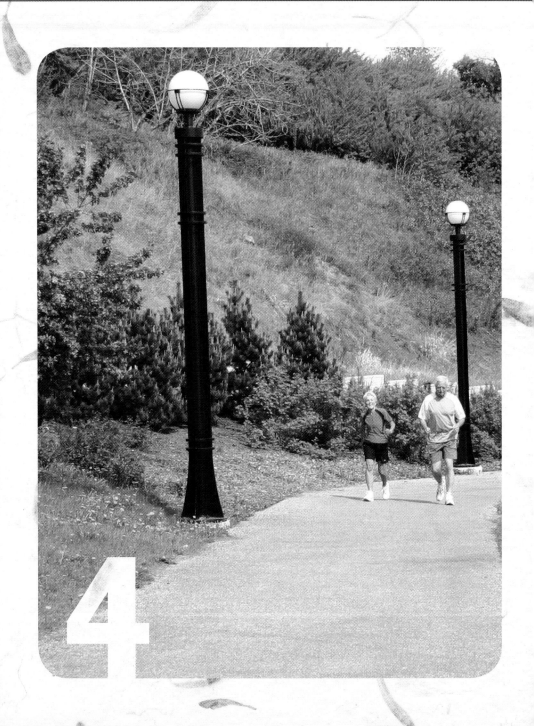

4

Introduction

Walking is suitable for most people regardless of age or fitness level. It's safe and improves your health with the least risk of injury to muscles and joints. Talk to your doctor before you start any exercise program.

Here Are Some Health Benefits You Can Look Forward to:

+ More energy
+ Less stress
+ Weight loss
+ Fewer aches and pains
+ Toned muscles
+ A healthier heart
+ Improved sleep
+ Improved self-esteem

Shoes and Socks

Like eye wear, shoe requirements are specific to each person. Get yourself fitted properly with a good pair of technical running shoes. The team at the Walking/Running Room is trained to fit you properly. Wear a pair of Double Layer™ socks. They are friction free, keep the feet drier and provide improved temperature control, to keep you warm in winter and cool in summer.

Clothes

At the Walking/Running Room you also will find fitness clothing that is weather-resistant and moves moisture away from your body. Wear clothes that are comfortable and appropriate for the season. Look for the Fit-Wear® brand of products.

Fall and Winter

Dress in layers. For above zero temperatures, wear a breathable jacket and a base layer against the skin. Below zero you'll need a hat, mitts and breathable jacket and pants. In addition, you will need long underwear made of a moisture-wicking material and an insulating polyester fleece layer for warmth.

Spring and Summer

Wear lightweight active wear made with performance fabrics. The Running Room Fit-Wear® brand of products is made of polyester fabric with a moisture-wicking treatment that enables sweat to move away from the body and evaporate. These clothes help keep you cool and dry and limit chafing.

Setting Your Goals

To get the most out of your training program, you should set an ultimate goal and then set several smaller goals to get you there. Your ultimate goal might be to walk a particular distance, but before you walk the distance you must first train consistently. It can help to set some smaller, shorter-distance targets to test you along the way. Interestingly, many athletic walkers will tell you that the true reward comes from the training, not the event itself.

Your goals can be qualitative or they can be quantitative: a qualitative long-term goal might be to make fitness part of your daily routine, just like brushing your teeth or combing your hair; a quantitative long-term goal might be to walk a specific event like the Terry Fox walk for cancer or to walk a half marathon to celebrate turning a new age.

Set short-term goals that allow you to savor some of your training rewards. Your first goal might be to walk continuously for 20 minutes. One good goal at the start of any program is to walk for 30 days without an injury, which will force you to listen to your body.

In Your Program, You Will Have Five Kinds of Goals:

1. A daily goal to get moving every day.

2. A self-acceptance goal to accept that daily fitness is part of your lifestyle.

3. A performance goal for a season—either a distance goal, such as walking a 5K, or a time goal, such as walking a specific distance in a specific time.

4. A dedication goal or a special goal for a season—something that will motivate you to continue training throughout the year. Dedicate your year to the memories of a loved one, or dedicate your goal to proving you can do it when others believe you cannot.

5. A dream goal—a big event, the achievement of a long-term weight goal or a special distance that seems just slightly out of reach but achievable.

If your goals are intelligent and realistic, you will be more likely to succeed and not get discouraged early in your training. There is no special formula for where you should start or the rate at which you should progress. Take care not to let your newfound fitness carry you past improvement into overuse. Don't look at the people around you. Look at where you are now and start a program of improvement from that point. Set a current benchmark and try to improve by approximately 10% a week. Keeping a limit of 10% a week allows you to improve while minimizing your risk of injury.

To help you along the way in both assessment and encouragement, start a log-book. A daily log will reinforce your progress towards your goals. There is a certain pleasure that comes from recording your workouts and assessing the quality of the effort. Record the distance you walked, where you walked and the type of walk (e.g., hill workout, long and slow, fast training). Include notes on how you felt, especially if your stress level was above normal, resting heart rate, weight and any extreme weather conditions.

Be sure to monitor and evaluate your training. Adjust your program and goals to your progress and the other facets of your life. Use your logbook to document any changes in your circumstances and the corresponding adjustments to your short-term and long-term goals. Now, changes are not free-ride tickets that let you out of training, but you should back off if conditions warrant. For example, if the weather becomes extremely hot, you must intelligently modify the program. If a busy work schedule leaves you tired, and you have bad walks on two consecutive days, you need to slow down or take an extra rest day. Listen to your body. It is the voice of reason.

Remember that sometimes your daily goal is a rest day. Rest is a good four-letter word that lets your body rebuild and get stronger. Sports medicine experts recommend 48 hours to recover from a hard workout, so it should be a scheduled part of every training program.

The setting of athletic goals, the discipline of following a regimented program towards specific goals and the recording of your progress will transfer over into the other parts of your life. Studies continue to prove that people who are physically active are more positive in their approach to challenges, have more energy and eat better. These added benefits and feelings of improved health are some of the reasons walkers become highly self-motivated over a period of time.

You Should Decide on a Strategy:

A. Determine Your Goals

Try to establish weekly goals for improvement. The more realistic the goals, the more likely you will not be discouraged partway through your training. Use a walking logbook to help evaluate your progress. Always be ready to readjust and reevaluate your goals. For example, bad walks on two consecutive days may indicate a need to back off and progress more slowly.

Short-term goals:

e.g., to complete a 5K charity walk
e.g., to lose 10 lb.

Long-term goals:

e.g., to lose 25 lb. and have fitness as a part of your daily routine
e.g., to walk a half marathon

Remember!

Your goals can be qualitative (e.g., to get in shape) or quantitative (e.g., walk a 45-minute 5K).

B. Record Your Goals

Commit to your goals by writing them down and review your progress towards these goals on an active basis.

C. Monitor Your Progress by Means of a Logbook

Logbooks reinforce your daily step-by-step progress towards achievement of goals.

D. Modify Your Goals

As you progress in your training, your short-term and even long-term goals may change. Modify your goals according to changes in circumstance and document this change.

Focus on aspects within your control, e.g., skills, preparation. Avoid outcome goals beyond your immediate control, e.g., scores, placing, winning.

How to Start:

Step 1

Write down a difficult but achievable ultimate goal. This goal is what you are striving to achieve overall.

LONG-TERM DREAM GOAL:

_____

_____

_____

_____

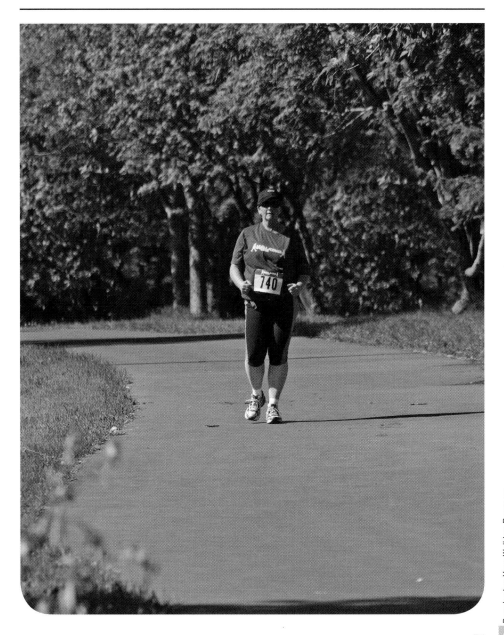

Step 2

Write down your dream goal for the next few months. This is a short-term goal that is still a great challenge and would normally be a step towards being able to achieve your ultimate goal. i.e., to complete a 10 km race while working towards a half marathon.

DREAM GOAL FOR THIS SEASON:

_____

_____

_____

_____

Step 3

Write down your realistic performance goal for this season. It might help to set dates for other goals leading to the performance goal, such as walking a distance within a certain time or completing a walking distance.

REALISTIC PERFORMANCE GOAL FOR THIS SEASON:

_____

_____

_____

_____

Step 4

Evaluate your progress and consider whether you are aiming too high (you might need more base mileage) or whether you should set yourself a harder target.

SELF-ACCEPTANCE GOAL:

_____

_____

_____

_____

Step 5

Establish a weekly goal for improvement. Remember that the more realistic you are, the better your chances of attaining your goal. Use a training log to record your progress. Use the *Running Room Training Log* to record how you feel and where you ran. Modify your training if necessary.

DAILY GOAL:

_____

_____

_____

_____

For some, walking a certain distance or time is reward enough. Others may want to lose a certain amount of weight, and yet others may want to competitive walk or race walk. Goals are personal to you—don't think about what others strive for. The best goal is to compete against ourselves.

Design Your Own Training Program

A. Strategy for the Development of a Training Program: Factors to Consider

1. How much time do you have? E.g., five days a week approximately, one hour/day, include prep time

2. How much of a commitment are you willing to make? E.g., four days a week for the first month and five days a week afterwards

3. Available facilities

4. Present level of fitness

5. Psychological demands, e.g., stress, anxiety, work, family and community demands

B. Designing Your Schedule

1. Decide on the distance or time that you wish to train relative to your goals. E.g., a 5K is the focus of many charitable walks.

2. Determine the number of walking days per week that will be needed and that you can commit to. Strive for at least three workouts per week.

3. Select the appropriate day of the week for each workout. Build in a hill walk, easy walk, long walk, rest and some alternate exercise.

4. Determine the total weekly distance goal you think you will be able to do. Refer to sample programs. Increase no more than 10% per week.

5. Determine the appropriate distance for each day's workout to equal your total weekly distance goal. You may split distance evenly, but it is usually easier to go hard/easy, and to alternate longer and shorter walks.

6. Record this plan in your *Running Room Training Log*.

7. Use a pedometer or Garmin device to monitor your distance walked, pace, calories burnt and heart rate.

C. Determining Weekly Distance

Determining the right amount of distance for the week can be difficult. Use the following tips to determine the distance level best suited to you.

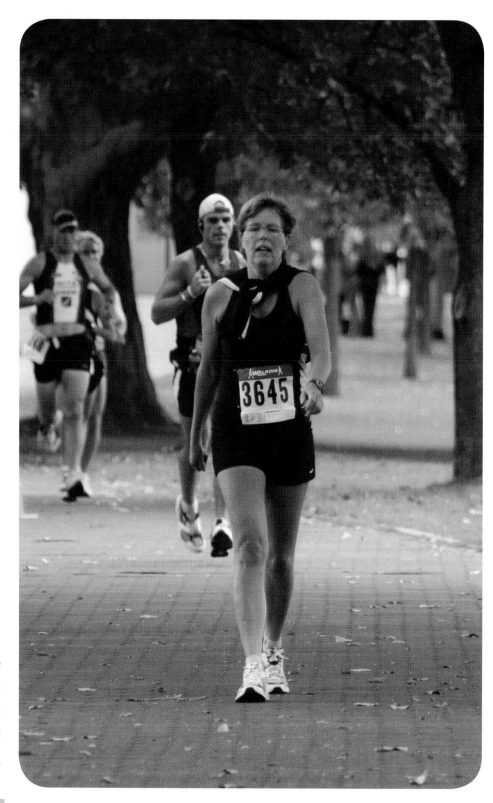

1. When is my free time and how much time is available? E.g., I have 45 minutes available at noon.

2. Are you starting out physically fit and injury free?

3. Are you mentally fit? E.g., motivated, charged or tired, depressed, etc.

* Depending on your responses, you may need to increase or decrease the distance or time you plan to walk for the week. Listen to your body. It is best to build up your distance gradually over a period of several months to avoid injury.

Training Rules

1. This program starts conservatively. You can even fall a little behind and still get back on the program.

2. Once you reach the halfway mark, you may find it difficult to keep up unless you walk faithfully at least three times a week.

3. If you can't keep up, or you lose time from illness or injury, don't panic. Stay at the level you can handle or go back a level until you are ready to move on.

4. Remember, it took you a lot of years to get out of shape; take your time getting back into shape. You will get back in shape much faster if you stay injury free.

Long Slow Distance Using a Combination of Walking and Strolling

Long slow distance walks are the cornerstone of this training program. They include brisk walking and strolling combinations. These sessions of stress while brisk walking and rest while strolling allow you to go farther and faster and recover better. Brisk walking is done at a pace you would walk if you were late for an appointment. Strolling is a pace you would do while window-shopping. Take a full minute to stroll for every 10 minutes of your brisk walk. You should feel a moderate increase in your breathing and start to perspire.

The long slow distances increase the capillary network in your body and raise your anaerobic threshold. They mentally prepare you for long distances.

Walking

Walking has been around for years in the history of sports and as a means of transport. However, walking as a choice in health and fitness was never really given the importance and stature of sports such as running, cycling or swimming. That has changed. Out of the running revolution, walking fitness has emerged as a viable alternative to running that provides the same benefits without the same level of risk and injury.

Walk or Run

Throughout history, mankind has walked and ran. The moderate effort corresponds wonderfully with the design of the body's aerobic system of energy production. The word "aerobic" has come to mean "with oxygen" to sport scientists and educators and now to millions of fitness enthusiasts. Our aerobic system works well, producing all the energy we require for the vast majority of our needs. As long as we take in enough oxygen with the air we breathe, the aerobic system functions as a miracle of conservation, recycling and efficiency.

In most cultures, running has been simply the body's emergency response system. This fight or flight response enables us to move much more quickly than our normal walk, but only for a short period of time. In their early days on earth, our ancestors used this system to escape from becoming lunch or to catch lunch.

Most of us have only about a minute of this high level of activity at our disposal. Trained athletes can stretch it out a little longer. We all know the heavy-legged feeling and stomach queasiness when we have reached our personal limit.

Physiologically, our body's oxygen-based operating system senses that we are not getting the fuel we need. A series of defense mechanisms rush to protect us: our breathing becomes labored; our muscles feel incapable of more effort. We have no choice but to slow down and stop—at best gasping for breath; at worst, feeling distinctly ill. Our fatigue is only the first in a series of defense mechanisms that nature has provided us with. It is cautioning us to slow down and to gradually build up intensity and distance.

It took many centuries for most of us to realize that we could manipulate our aerobic system to allow us to walk or run long distances without stopping. This is called training. Training programs have grown more intelligent, allowing more people to discover their athletic capabilities.

What's the Difference Between Walking and Running?

Both running and walking have much to offer, including maximum health benefits and truly life-altering experiences.

The primary difference between walking and running: walking takes longer. Yes, big surprise. While it does require a bigger investment in time, walkers sustain far fewer injuries.

Walking is a gentle option for many athletes. The impact force of walking is little more than the body weight you carry just by standing upright. Now you can handle that. So, let's walk!

Fitness Walking Benefits

Cardiovascular Fitness

The regular activity of walking for as little as 25–30 minutes will increase the efficiency of your heart and lungs and boost your ability to perform other tasks with less fatigue.

Muscular Endurance

Muscular endurance allows you to exercise for a longer period of time without undue fatigue in the working muscles. Increased muscular endurance is a natural result of an exercise program with repeated, low-intensity actions. Walking is an ideal form of this type of exercise.

Muscular Strength

Walkers build strength in the muscles they use as they walk. These muscles are primarily in the legs, hips and buttocks. In power walking and race walking techniques, strength is also acquired in the muscles of the upper back, chest and shoulders. Walkers sometimes begin a further program of strength training in the gym to develop and complement the strength they gain from walking. This, in turn, enhances the duration, the speed and the efficiency of the walking itself.

Walkers land with a force equivalent to only 1–1.5 times body weight. This is much less than a runner whose landing force can be equivalent to 3–4 times one's body weight. The stress on the bones and joints is therefore much reduced and many common injuries associated with running are almost eliminated.

Walking is a weight-bearing activity and therefore helps the bones stay strong. Walking is accepted as an activity that prevents or reduces the effects of osteoporosis, because it builds and maintains bone density.

In addition to helping with the maintenance of a healthy weight, or to lose weight if you need to, walking manages stress, keeps you more positive and allows you to sleep better.

Immune System

Exercise in general stimulates the immune system. It is well established that those exercising consistently at a moderate intensity tend to get sick less.

Blood Pressure

Walking will lower high blood pressure or keep normal blood pressure on target.

Breast Cancer

A study published in the *Journal for Breast Cancer Research* documented that active women had about a 13% lower risk of postmenopausal breast cancer.

Body Composition

Walking tones and builds the muscles. Because muscle tissue is heavier than fat, you may not actually lose weight by exercise. (Nor will your fat "convert" to muscle!) However, you are very likely to lose fat at the same time as you gain muscle. As you begin to lose the fat, you will notice how toned your muscles have become. You feel and look like an athlete.

Self-Esteem

There are many studies and loads of incidental information that exercise improves our energy levels and our personal self-esteem! As a walker you soon feel strong and fit and in control of both your athletic and personal goals.

Types of Fitness Walking

What's in a Name?

In this book fitness walking is the name we have given to all the various types of walking. Under the fitness walking umbrella, we use three other names to describe the forms of walking that interest most participants.

We have chosen **active walking** to describe the normal way in which we get around on two feet. We define it as normal walking that is done as a fitness and lifestyle choice. Active walking can be an introduction to increased fitness or a wonderful means to take you around the lake or around the world.

We use **power walking** to describe walking that is adapted to provide a more dynamic form of exercise than active walking. When you power walk, you are

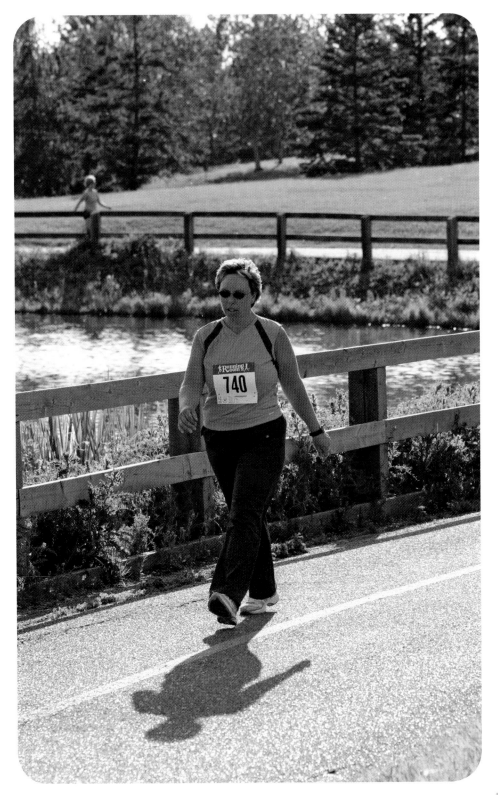

definitely aiming for a workout. You are prepared to put some effort into the activity and do your walking with purpose.

We use the term **athletic walking** for walking at a faster pace with more intensity. We sometimes use it interchangeably with race walking because race walking is one form of athletic walking.

We use race walking to describe walking with the effort one uses in a race. It is aided by the excitement of the crowd, other walkers and the thrill of the finish line. You do not have to race although we can tell you what is involved if you are interested. But when you learn race walking technique, you will be doing the fastest walking there is. As a fitness walker, you'll get a great workout. The activity can become quite intense if you choose to pick up the pace. Even if you have no intention of competing, with race walking, you may never miss an appointment again.

Various names have appeared over the years to describe walking activities. We're not sure what some of them exactly mean. Some may be clever labels to make various systems commercially attractive. Others may merely be ways to avoid the word "race," as in race walking. Race walkers are actually proud of the name. They know that the phrase just refers to the style of walking that is used in races. Many people are frightened by race walking technique and style. They fear embarrassment, and they resist trying the sport.

Active Walking

Active walking is the term we use in this program for normal walking. But for us, it's normal walking done as a lifestyle choice.

Active walking can be the beginning of a fitness program or the fulfillment of a goal. If, for whatever reason, you have been sedentary for some time, even a short walk may be your first step on the road back to fitness. Fear of embarrassment keeps many of us from starting a fitness program. Running the first time through your neighborhood can be embarrassing. However, walk through your neighborhood and you discover no one really pays any attention to you. They just think you are out for an enjoyable walk.

No time? We can all relate, but the commitment to make time is actually your biggest fitness decision in these early stages. Everything else falls naturally into place. Walking does not have to involve a special trip to the club. It is just as much a fitness activity when it's part of your daily schedule.

Walk to the store for the newspaper or the milk. Walk the kids to school. Walk to work, at least partway. Park a few blocks away, or get off the bus a stop or two before your normal one. Decide to walk up and down a few flights of stairs in the office.

Be positive and creative in assessing what you're accomplishing. If it takes you 30 minutes to walk 3 kilometers to work and 15 minutes to drive and park, you are only using 15 minutes of additional time. Your 3 km training session has really only taken 15 minutes out of your day! Not only a solid workout, it also demonstrates great time management.

Active walking elevates your heart rate to an adequate level to provide a safe, moderate training effect for your heart, lungs and blood circulation. Equally important, walking uses particular muscles that contribute to your most efficient posture. If your aches and pains result from underused muscles, you may well find the twinges going away by themselves. People may begin to comment that you seem taller or look fitter. Enjoy the compliments.

You will certainly break the vicious circle of a less active lifestyle. Other activities will now be within your grasp, and less of a chore than they were previously.

Once active walking is part of your routine, your horizon is as wide as you choose to make it. Maybe you will choose to walk all the way to work. Maybe your holidays will be so much more enjoyable because you can walk around Vancouver's Sea Wall, Old Montreal or the Chicago Waterfront. Walking will become the holiday itself, as your walks evolve naturally into invigorating and fulfilling sightseeing hikes.

In this program you will learn how walking works and what it can do for you. You will better understand the way in which your body works. You will learn how comfortable shoes and clothing, good exercise habits and proper nutrition help your walking. You will be introduced to two other forms of walking that build on the momentum you have gained. Once you hit your stride with active walking, there are bigger and faster strides that you can take if you choose.

Power Walking

The term power walking suggests strong, dynamic action. There are no rules, no specific requirements, no referees and no penalties. Power walking simply adds effort to active walking with the aim of increasing the pace and physical demands of the activity. This, in turn, produces greater fitness benefits. I like to

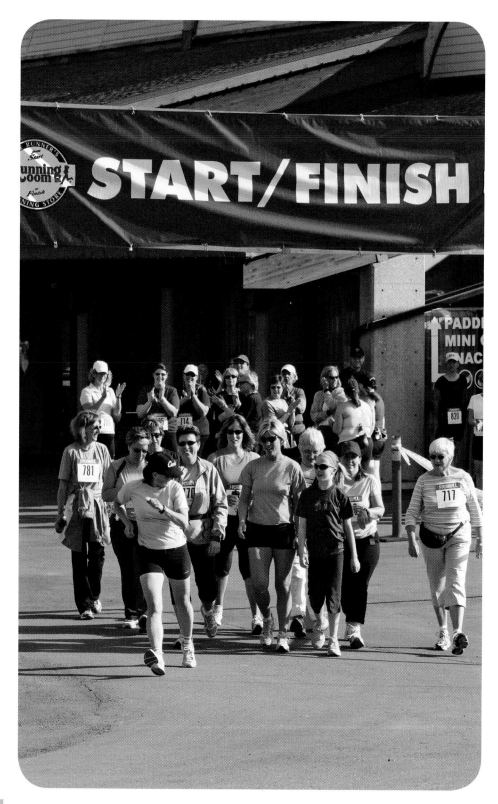

think of power walking as "I am late for my appointment" walking, where we notice our breathing and feel our perspiration.

Power walkers move with deliberate and slightly exaggerated movements. Strides are longer and our arms swing dynamically. A whole new level of fitness can be developed as you continue to walk with a purpose.

Because of its dynamic nature, power walking is often faster than active walking, but speed is not the ultimate objective. The idea is to extend the fitness benefits of regular walking by introducing additional muscular actions.

Power walking elevates your heart rate to a higher level than active walking, but avoids the high impact of other activities. Cardiovascular capacity and strength are improved. Your normal postural muscles are used to a greater degree.

In this program, you will be invited to try power walking. We will also introduce you to structured training sessions and show you how to design your own.

Athletic Walking

You don't have to race! But you will be able to if you feel the competitive urge. Athletic walking is a natural evolution of active walking. It's the name given to the techniques used by those who do compete. Quite simply, it's the fastest you can go and still be walking. Competitive race walking can really test your level of fitness.

In our introduction to power walking, actions are added to regular walking in order to increase the effort and therefore the fitness benefits.

Race walking does the opposite. The technique takes away those elements of normal walking that slow us down. Our walking gets smoother and quicker, much quicker. The real fitness benefits come from the increased effort caused by the higher speed. If you are looking to reach the level of high intensity while avoiding extra pounding, athletic walking is for you.

In races, walkers have to observe two simple rules of technique, which have stood the test of time for well over 100 years. We will be teaching you those rules too. Of course, you won't have judges watching you on your daily walks. But the fact is, the rules define a technique, which is more efficient and ultimately faster. You'll find that working on your technique will make your walking look and feel better. If you're in the vast majority, you will improve with practice. In the meantime, just get out and walk. The fitness benefits are there for everyone.

If you decide that you want to go in a judged race at some stage, you'll need to make sure that your technique will keep the judges happy. You'd do the same in a golf tournament or a tennis match.

In this program, you will learn and practice the basics of athletic race walking technique. The emphasis will be to find your target rhythm, which is the highest speed at which you can comfortably race walk. At that point, training sessions will be designed to use that rhythm to improve your endurance, coordination and strength. An introduction to the structure of a typical race walk competition will be provided for those who are interested.

Walk Before You Race

Many people ask about walking programs. They ask because they are remembering the running they enjoyed before the kids came along. Very often, they don't think they could run again because their knee, back or ankle injury would flair up if they tried. For many people, walking is an intelligent option.

If there are no specific medical problems that rule out activity in your particular case, we may be able to help. These days doctors prefer people to be active. They get surgery patients back on their feet as soon as it is safe to do so. They will certainly encourage you to exercise unless there is a real medical reason why you should not.

Doctors do this to address the similar problems that took you out of action in the first place. The body works on the principle of if you don't use it, you lose it. If you are not training, you are de-training. Anyone forced to take time off experiences how quickly we lose our fitness. In a period of 30 days much of your fitness is lost. Your muscles lose their tone, your connective tissue may not be as tough and even your bones may have lost strength. You get caught in a vicious circle.

This may sound depressing, but understanding the problem is the key to solving it. You are all athletes; some of you are just at a lower level of fitness than you once were. This book will show you how to awaken the athlete hidden within. You remember what you can do. With some patience and intelligent training, we will walk you back to a fit and athletic life.

Walking virtually eliminates the many strenuous actions of other sports. The action, which causes so many problems in other sports, is the landing impact on each stride. The eccentric muscle contractions needed to hold you up require a degree of strength in the muscle, which you have lost to a greater or lesser extent.

Your fitness is not really lost. It's there—you just haven't used it for a while. I will help you find it so you can return you to an active lifestyle. This walking program can help you get it back. You've heard of high impact and low impact activities. Walking is a low impact sport, and it is a gentle yet progressive way to get the muscles working again.

Go through this program with the idea that you are training to be athletic. You may evaluate your progress by the amount of effort required to cover a distance. Patience is part of this program—with time and commitment you will see some major improvements.

Watch your anti-gravity muscles quietly respond to your walking routine. Don't be surprised if the old knee, back or ankle injury gives you a little less trouble than expected. Often, a regular range of motion helps in the debilitating effect of old injuries. We will show you how to balance the right amount of activity into your walking program to reap the maximum benefits.

The Walking Room Training Principles: Progressive Overload

Walking seems to attract hardworking, goal-oriented people who appreciate the fact that the sport rewards honest effort. These individuals have learned that the more they put in, the more they get out. Walking is different. Your willpower and your heart-lung machinery can handle much more work than your muscu-lo-skeletal system. Beyond a certain point, it's better to relax about your training than to approach every workout in hyper drive. The following guidelines show you how you can safely enjoy your walking without risking injury.

1. Honestly Evaluate Your Fitness Level

If you haven't had a physical exam lately, have one before you begin your walking program. Start out walking gently and slow to a stroll when you feel tired. Remember: You should be able to carry on a conversation as you walk. If you're patient with yourself, you can increase your effort as your body builds strength and adapts to the stress of walking.

2. Easy Does It

The generally accepted rule for increasing your distance is to edge upward no more than 10% per week. Beginner walkers should add just 1 or 2 kilometers per week to their totals. This amount doesn't sound like too much, but it will help keep you healthy, and that means you can continue building.

3. Plan for Plateaus

Don't increase your distance every week. Build to a comfortable level and then plateau there to let your body adjust. For example, you might build to a total walking time of 100 weekly minutes (walking fitness beginner level program, page 271) or a total distance of 21K per week (half marathon beginner training program, page 312). Stay at that training level for two to three weeks before gradually increasing again. Another smart tactic is to scale back periodically. On page 115 you will see an example of a 10-week conditioning program where there are adaptation weeks when the volume drops back. Don't allow yourself to get caught up by the thrill of increasing your distance every single week. That simply can't work very long.

4. Make Haste Slowly

Another cause of injury and fatigue is increasing the speed of your training walks too much and too often. The same is true of interval workouts, hill walking and race walking. When the time is right for faster paced walking (after you're completely comfortable with the amount of training you're doing), ease into it just once a week. Never do fast walking more than twice a week. Balance your fast workouts and your long walks (both "hard" days) with slower, shorter days. This is the well-known and widely followed hard-easy training system.

5. Strive for Efficient Walking Form

You'll have more fun because you won't be struggling against yourself. We will cover proper form in later chapters, but good posture is the core of walking technique and form. Posture is the result of muscles working in the way in which nature intended. Keep your head up: look in front of you, not down. Relax your shoulders and neck muscles. Walk tall by gently contracting the stomach muscles and the gluteus (the cheeks of your butt). Tilt the pelvis slightly, tucking it under your body and allowing the hips to move the legs forward more easily and with improved alignment.

6. Turn Away from Fad Diets: Go Instead with Wholesome Foods

Walkers function best on a diet high in complex carbohydrates. That means eating plenty of fruits, vegetables, whole-grain products and low-fat dairy foods and avoiding fried foods, pastries, cookies, ice cream and other fat-laden items. Fish, lean meats and poultry are better for you than high-fat sausage, bacon, untrimmed red meats and cold cuts. Generally, you're wise to eat three to four hours before walking. That way, you're less likely to experience bloating or nausea. Remember: fluids are vital. Aim to drink 8 to 10 glasses of water a day.

7. Hills

Hills place an enormous stress on the cardiovascular system, so it's best to warm up for several miles so you raise your heart rate gradually. When walking hills, shorten your stride and concentrate on lifting your knees and landing on the heel and rolling more on the front of your foot. Pump your arms like a cross-country skier. Lean forward but keep your back straight, your hips in, your chest out and your head up. Barreling down a steep hill can multiply skeletal forces several fold, which increases chances of injury. Hold your arms low and tilt your body forward to keep it perpendicular to the slope. Allow your stride to stretch out a little, but don't exaggerate it. Try to avoid the breaking action of landing too hard on your heels.

8. Be Smart About Injuries

Walkers who interrupt their training programs at the first sign of injury generally recover very quickly. You might not be able to enter the race you're aiming for, but you'll be able to find another one soon. On the other hand, walkers who persist in training hard even after they start to break down are courting much more serious injuries. When you develop a persistent walking pain, open your eyes and obey the red flag. Stop, rest and wait until your body is ready to begin training again. When it is, ease back into your training. Don't try to catch up too quickly: it can't be done.

9. Pay Close Attention to Pain

It's usually OK to forget mild discomfort if it goes away during a walk and doesn't return after. But pain that worsens during a walk or that returns after each walk cannot be ignored. Remember: pain has a purpose. It's a warning sign from your body that something's wrong. Don't overlook it. Instead, change your walking pattern, or if the pain is severe enough, stop walking and seek professional help.

"Any Pain, No Brain"

Biomechanics

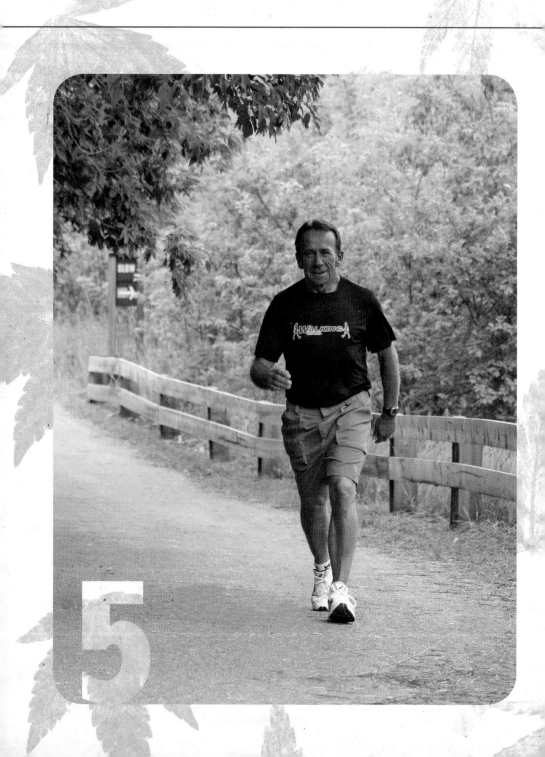

5

Walking Form

The Foot Plant

Our feet and gait are a gift from our parents. However, there are some things you can control and some you cannot. First, let your shoe professional at the Walking/Running Room fit you with a couple of pairs of shoes that meet your specific need. Once done, let's start walking and have fun.

In a normal stride there is a defined sequence of actions. The foot lands marginally on the outside of the heel before the rest of the sole rolls naturally forward before giving a final push with the ball of the foot. The first part of the stride tends to be slightly on the outside of the foot, with a roll inwards towards the end of the stride. This action is called pronation.

Your personal stride is the result of your shape, physique, and strength and balance of your muscles. Much of these are genetically passed on from your parents. For some of us with athletic parents, this is a blessing. For others whose parents were card players and TV fans, we must work a little harder, but the results will be worth the effort. Please don't try to change your foot plant as you train. You will not be walking naturally, and you are very likely to sustain an injury. Changes to your gait only happen as a result of longer term changes elsewhere.

As you gain fitness and strength, you may well notice that many irregularities resolve themselves. Modern training shoes are designed to accommodate biomechanical variances in the walker's feet. Often a problem you thought you had will turn out to be not much of a problem after all. But if you really do have a problem that continues to affect your activity, you may have to seek the advice of a therapist, physician or coach to assess and deal with your particular situation. They should be part of your success team.

Stride Rate, Not Stride Length

Studies show as walkers get faster, their stride length actually decreases, but the stride rate, called turnover rate, increases. Too long a stride results in three problems.

In an athletically efficient gait the foot is already moving backwards when it hits the ground. When our foot is stuck out in front of us, we slow down the forward momentum.

Secondly, too long a stride will land at a point ahead of the body's center of mass.

It's like putting on a brake; we have to wait until our foot is directly under the body before we start pushing forward again. Shorten the stride and we land more under our body and our momentum carries us forward.

Thirdly, extra time in the air is largely wasted. When our feet aren't on the ground, they're not driving us forward. Unless you are naturally endowed with a long stride, that is already efficient, improvements in your own personal efficiency are likely to come first from shortening your stride. Lengthening your stride naturally is a long-term process of increased fitness and muscle strengthening.

Overstriding works the muscles harder than they need to. They will tighten up and tire before your walk is done. The fatigue will make you soon revert to your natural stride length anyway.

Practice Your Technique

Once or twice a week, a little technique work is really helpful. After your warm-up, walk some accelerations of 50–150 meters. Pick one of the elements of good form and feel yourself executing it well during the acceleration. Rehearse each element at least four times, and keep to one or two elements at most in each session. A change in technique may feel a little awkward at first, but as your coordination and skill improves, it feels good. We are designed to walk fast.

You can also follow the lead of athletes in events like sprinting and hurdling where effective technique is a vitally important ingredient of their success. The warm-up is actually designed so that athletes' technique or skill is rehearsed every time they prepare for training or competition.

Your warm-up already consists of a period of walking and stretching. Build in some technique and form accelerations. Your motor skills improve most by focusing on one point of technique for a short period of time and then repeating it several times.

In technique and form work, the short periods are the key. When you're moving your body in a new way, your brain literally tires quite quickly! You'll feel it happen. There will be a noticeable but temporary loss in your coordination. It's temporary; the short break between accelerations will give you the recovery you need. Keep the high-quality session short to maintain form and coordination. You only want to practice good form not bad form.

The Basics of Athletic Walking Technique

Race walking is the fastest and is designed for speed. There is a clear transition from regular walking to race walking. The leisurely low effort aspects of walking are replaced with dynamic, highly efficient actions. These result in trained athletes being able to reach speeds of over 15 kilometers per hour while observing the rules of race walking.

Feet, Ankles and Knees

Feet are placed directly in front of each other in an attempt to progress in as straight a line as possible. Any slight outward turn of the foot loses a couple of centimeters on each stride. The ankle and knee flexion of regular walking replaces the jaunty bounce of a purposeful stroll. It is done with a much greater degree of control provided by the strong contractions of the leg muscles.

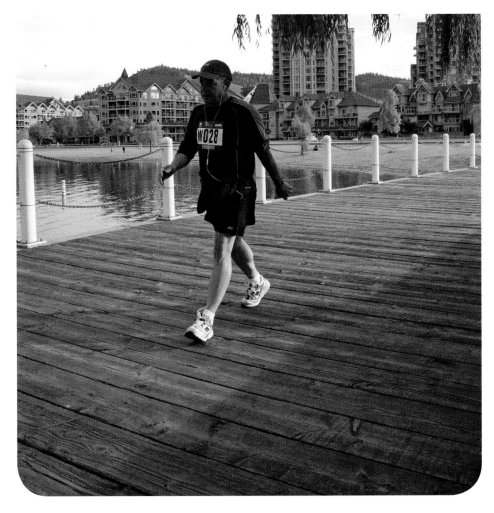

Hip

Perhaps one of the most unique and recognizable actions of race walkers are the hips moving forward and down, not side to side. Race walkers are driven, and appear to wiggle. The motions accomplish the following:

1. The forward motion increases the length of each stride without any side-to-side lateral motion, which slows the stride rate. Race walkers use the hip to carry the whole body into an advantageous position to begin the next drive. The advancing foot strikes the ground almost directly below the center of mass. More importantly, the foot is already moving backwards. Without the hip action, the foot lands ahead of the center of mass, resulting in the braking action, which has to be overcome before the next drive phase.

2. The dropping of each hip provides the action, which is often misinterpreted as a wiggle. The hip opposite to the locked supporting leg drops. This allows the body's center of mass to move forward without the need to rise up over the straight supporting leg. The whole body moves forward more smoothly with wasted motion avoided.

Although the hip action is a distinctive feature of race walking, it does not define it. Even the best walkers vary greatly in hip mobility and use. Effective hip action certainly lengthens and flattens the stride. But if attempting a classic hip movement slows your rhythm, don't worry. Fast, efficient rhythm is more important than a slower technique, however classic. The modification of hip action will be a longer-term project improving with practice.

Arms

The arms are bent at the elbow, creating this shorter lever. This shorter lever creates faster movement. The arm action is dynamic for middle distance walking and helps to provide a fast turnover rate.

The arms swing forward and back, with lateral motion reduced as much as possible. Upward movement at the end of the forward arm swing should also be avoided, because the effect is to lift the body. Walking is about forward motion with a minimal amount of vertical motion.

Race walking is the exception to the elbow-at-90-degrees rule on the arms. Race walkers want to go in the shortest and straightest line possible from start to finish. The key is to keep the forearm as parallel to the ground as reasonably possible. This will mean that the elbow angle opens a little when the arm is in front of the body and closes a little when it is behind. Imagine your arms working like pistons to drive you forward.

The arms do not actually drive you forward, but the rhythm of their action does reflect the stride rhythm and leg turnover rate. So you can use your arm action as a cue to remind your legs of the rate of turnover. The legs will match a short and quick arm action. Use your body's lateral mid-line as a guide. Don't take your hand behind the mid-line as the arm moves back and don't take the elbow in front of the mid-line as the arm drives forward.

Fatigue, caused by the dynamic motion, may result in hunched shoulders, pulling the arm carriage up high. This position is inefficient, and it also has the effect of raising the center of mass, which contributes to lifting and wasted energy. The hands should be low enough to almost brush the hips on each swing. This low arm carriage is achieved by keeping the shoulders relaxed. Newton's law also applies: With every action there is a reaction; the arms drive back and your legs drive forward.

Overall Body Position

Your body should be upright. The tendency to lean forward has three significant effects. First, there is a considerable loss of the power generated by the arms. Second, stride length is reduced. Third, lifting may occur as the rear foot is pulled prematurely off the ground.

Forward lean is often a result of fatigue. A backward lean is less common and is likely caused by a weakness or imbalance in the postural muscles. Correction is therefore longer term, but attention is warranted because of the undoubted loss of a portion of the drive phase.

Rhythm

The ability to maintain rhythm is the key to race walking success. Muscular endurance through regular training at a target rhythm is a theme running through our training program. The other components of stamina, strength and speed are all linked together and defined by the ability to maintain rhythm for the appropriate race distance. We'll deal with this important idea in the sections for more advanced walkers.

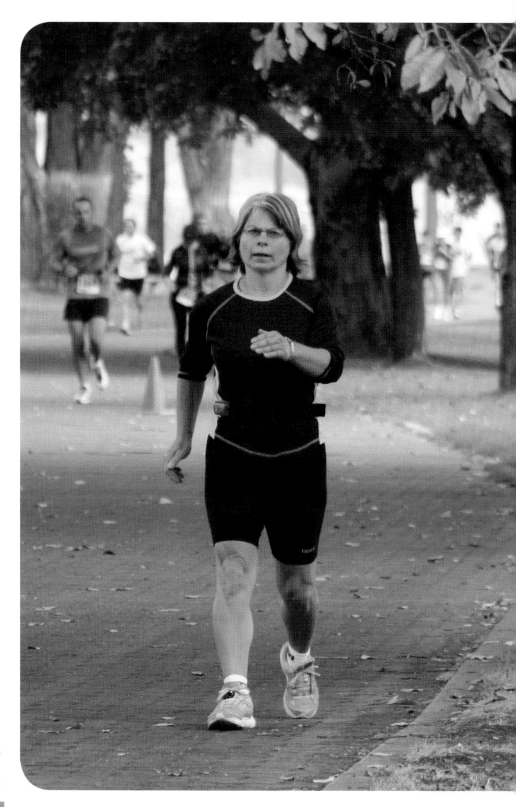

Walking Form Checklist

Posture

1. Is your posture erect?

☐ Walk tall—shoulders and chest up and open. Keep your head level and look forward, not down. Glance down to monitor your step, but keep your chin up.

☐ Relax your neck, back and shoulders.

Chest and Hips

2. Is your chest open? Are your hips moving forward?

☐ Chest out—shoulders back. Pull back your shoulders and open the chest for improved posture. Dropping your shoulders closes off the chest, restricting your breathing and limiting your arm motion.

☐ Your hips move forward and do not wiggle side to side.

Arm Action and Position

3. Are your arms loose at your side or at 90-degree angles?

☐ Bend your elbows at right angles swinging your arms faster—faster arm motion allows for faster walking.

☐ Swing your arms from shoulder and keep your elbows close to your body. Allow your hands to come to the center line of your body, but not to cross it in front.

☐ Cup your hands lightly to avoid clenching your fists. Imagine you are gently holding soda crackers.

Foot Strike and Push Off

4. Do you feel your foot roll smoothly from heel to toe?

☐ As you step forward, lift your toes and plant the heel of your lead foot. Roll through the entire foot and push off with your toes, lifting your heel high. Feel your foot roll smoothly from heel to toe.

☐ Avoid overstriding and bouncing. Walking is all forward motion.

☐ Count your stride rate—walking faster generally requires faster steps. I will provide a basic guideline to follow, which allows you to compare your steps per minute to approximate speed, pace and effort.

Proper Shoe Selection

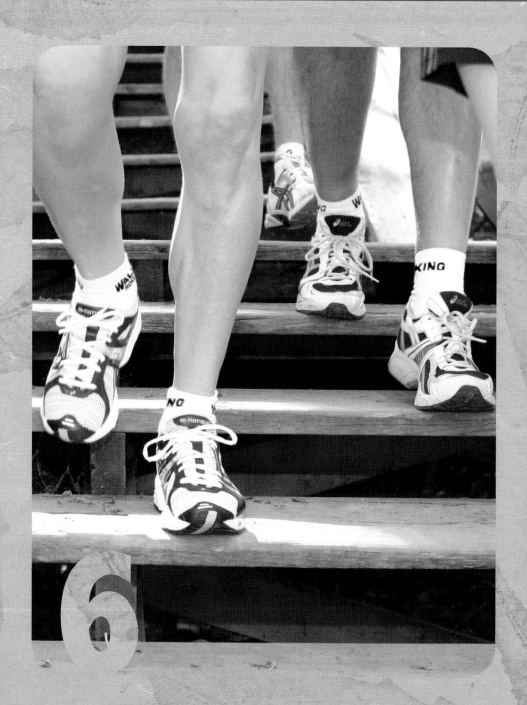

6

Overview

Finding the right pair of shoes—the ones that give you the best fit, comfort and support for the conditions in which you walk—is the best investment of both time and resources you can spend on yourself. Shoes are the most important piece of equipment. The average walker strikes the ground close to 1000 times every kilometer, or over 1700 times each mile, with forces close to three times their body weight. This weight has to be absorbed by the feet and legs, so it is important you put some thought into which pair you choose. The right pair of shoes can enhance your performance and prevent injuries.

Proper Shoe Selection

Proper shoe selection is an important part of the prevention of injury. Forces close to three times your body weight are placed on your feet and dissipate up through your leg when you walk. The right category of walking shoes will accommodate your individual needs and can keep you walking comfortably and hopefully injury free.

Determining Your Foot Type

After your heel initially strikes the ground, your foot ideally should pronate slightly by rolling inward and your arch starts to absorb the load and may start to flatten out. Your foot then supinates, which means it rotates outward after the weight is transferred to the ball of your foot. The foot in effect then becomes a rigid lever so that you propel yourself forward. Perfect walking styles are rare. Within the footstrike there will be varying degrees of pronation and supination. Natural pronation is more common than supination.

The Overpronator

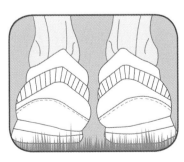

+ feet roll inward too much when walking
+ generally has low arches
+ knees move towards the medial or inside of the feet when you bend at the knees
+ more susceptible to iliotibial band syndrome, tendonitis, plantar fasciitis and patello-femoral syndrome

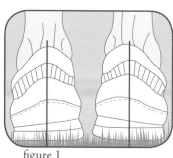

+ lacks normal medial or inward rolling of feet when walking
+ generally has high arches
+ knees move laterally or towards the outside of the feet when you bend at the knees
+ more susceptible to ankle sprains, stress fractures, pain on the outside of the shin and knee and plantar fasciitis

figure 1

Reading Old Shoes

Your old shoes reveal many traits about what type of walker you are. If you visit a Walking/Running Room to buy a new pair of walking shoes, a salesperson can often put you into the right pair in a matter of moments. Most magicians would never reveal the secrets of their trade, but I can take some of the mystery out of shoe selection with a few tips on how to read your old shoes.

View the Upper of the Shoe from the Rear:

+ The shoe's center line on the back of the heel counter (see figure 1 above) should be perpendicular to the ground.
+ The center line shifts severely inward, to the medial side of the shoe, if the walker has overpronated.
+ The center line shifts outward, to the lateral side of the shoe, if the walker has supinated.

Check the Condition of the Midsoles:

+ The midsole compresses uniformly if the walker has normal pronation.
+ The midsole compresses more on the inside of the shoe if the walker has overpronated.
+ The midsole compresses more on the outside of the shoe, if the walker has supinated.

Check the Wear on the Upper:

+ The upper retains its shape if the walker has normal pronation and during the propulsion phase, toes off—leaves the ground—in a neutral position.

Shoe Requirements and Support Features

The Overpronator Category

+ straight or semi-curved last is best
+ maximum rear-foot stability and has external heel counter for added support

- maximum cushioning at heel strike area
- substantial extended medial midsole support

The Stability Category
- semi-curved last
- moderate pronation guidance
- excellent cushioning at heel strike area
- durable, multidensity midsole material

The Neutral Category
- curved or semi-curved last is best
- low or moderate rear-foot to mid-foot stability
- flexible midsoles
- additional cushioning in midsole

Guidelines to Find the Best Shoe Fit
- Shop in the afternoon to get the right fit.
- Try on both shoes with the same type of sock to be worn during the activity.
- Try on several different models to make a good comparison.
- Walk around the store in the shoes.
- Check the quality of the shoes. Look at the stitching, eyelets and gluing. Feel for bumps inside the shoe.
- The sole should flex only where your foot flexes—across your metatarsal area.
- Your toes should not be pressing against the end of the shoe when standing nor should there be too much room. Shoes too big or too small can cause injury to the toenails while walking.
- The heel counter should fit snugly, so that there is very little slipping at the heel.
- Shoes should be comfortable on the day you buy them. Don't rely on a break-in period.
- Consult the staff at the Walking Room/Running Room for help in selecting the correct shoe.

Terms Used by Shoe Manufacturers
Arch Support
Refers to the inside portion of the shoe directly below the arch of the foot. Most shoes don't have a separate arch support unless it is attached to the removable insole.

Strobel Stitch Lasting

A new and widely accepted method of stitching the upper of the shoe onto the outer edge of a soft and pliable material, which resembles the shape of the insole. This is then attached to the midsole. The advantage of this method is to provide a softer, lighter and more flexible footbed while providing some torsional rigidity.

Combination Lasting

A combination of two techniques—board lasting and slip lasting—for joining the upper, last and midsole of a shoe. Usually the back of the shoe is board-lasted for stability while the front is slip-lasted for flexibility. This combination gives stability in the rear-foot with flexibility and cushioning in the forefoot.

Slip Lasting

A technique for joining the upper, last and midsole of a shoe. The upper of the shoe is placed over the last and sewn together at the bottom, similar to a moccasin. It's then attached to the midsole. Slip-lasted shoes have no boards to cause stiffness. On the other hand, they are less stable than board-lasted shoes.

Curve-Lasted

Refers to the curvature of a shoe. Curve-lasted shoes have an angle between the rear foot and the forefoot. Most people have moderately curved feet, and shoe companies work with lasts curved about seven degrees. This is comfortable for most walkers. The average walker should stay away from severely curved shoes, which can cramp and blister the toes and forefoot.

Straight-Lasted

As with the term curve-lasted, straight-lasted refers to the curvature of a shoe. A straightlasted shoe is constructed on a last with no curve. Theoretically, the shoe could almost be worn on either foot. Straight-lasted shoes are perfectly adequate for most walkers and clearly the best selection for walkers with flat feet.

External Heel Counter Stabilizers

Supports that keep the heel counter from breaking down or away from the midsole under stress. They're usually designed to help control excessive rear foot motion, and nearly all of the better made motion-control shoes have some heel counter support.

Heel Counter

Light, strong thermal plastic material that is firmly attached to the rear base of the shoe. An extended heel counter that runs along the medial (inside) edge of the shoe will increase stability and reduce foot pronation and rotation.

Insoles

Also called sockliners. These line the inside bottom of a shoe and are often removable. If a shoe doesn't come with a good smooth one, replace the insole with whatever insert you need for healthy walking.

Last

The basic form on which a shoe is built. This provides a sculpted profile, which resembles an anatomically correct representation of the foot. Many shoes are now made for specific genders because men and women require different configurations.

Midsole Density

Relates to the firmness of the midsole. A multidensity midsole has materials of different firmness in strategic locations, which can be a big advantage to walkers with certain gait patterns. For example, a heavy pronator needs cushioning where the heel strikes but still needs firmness for stability when the foot starts to roll inward. With a multidensity midsole, the lateral (outer) part of the shoe, where the heel strikes, is soft for shock absorption, and the medial (inner) side is firm for increased stability.

Outsoles

Outsoles are the undersurface of a shoe that makes contact with the ground. Outsoles can be divided into two major categories: Either more aggressive (lugged) or more sculptured and road friendly. If you're going to be walking on dirt, loose gravel or grass trails, the more lugged outsole shoe provides excellent traction. The more road-friendly sole is better suited for asphalt or cement. The longer-lasting material has more carbonized blown rubber in the outsole, but it will add a little more weight. Along with added flex grooves, the rubber helps the rubber heel to toe transition and gives you the smoothest and most durable ride.

Uppers

The top covering of a shoe is a combination of mesh nylon, synthetic leather or suede. This is the best material for the uppers because it puts very little abrasive forces on the foot and allows it to breathe. Walkers who predominately exercise on trails have many choices in combinations of mesh nylon with leather and suede uppers. They are also reinforced at the toe with bumpers for added protection. Some shoes will come with waterproofing and weather-resistant materials, which help keep the foot dry and comfortable in wet or snow and cold conditions.

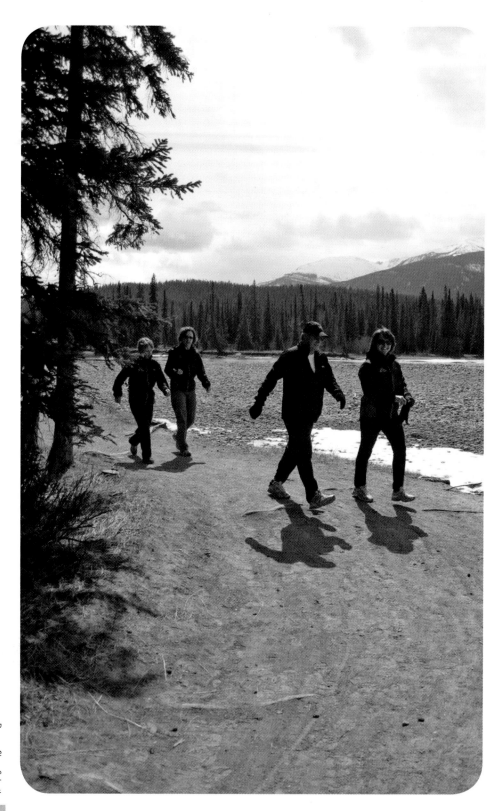

Three Categories of Walking Shoes

1. Support Shoes

You tend to break down midsoles over time, pronate to overpronate and need a firm midsole with a sturdy heel counter.

Guidance Features

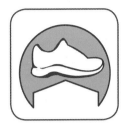

- straight or semi-curved last
- excellent rear-foot stability
- variable degree of extended medial support
- supportive and more rounded heel crash pad area

2. Cushioning Shoes

You need a well-cushioned shoe with a flexible forefoot with no medial guidance features.

Cushioning Features

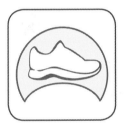

- curved last
- low or moderate rear-foot stability
- softer midsoles
- additional cushioning in midsole
- supportive and more rounded heel crash pad area

3. Rugged Walk/Trail Shoes

You require a stable shoe for uneven or loose trails. You need a more durable outsole.

Rugged Walk Features

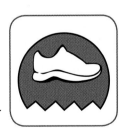

- aggressive lugged outsole
- toe bumper for protection
- forefoot protection plate—prevents stone bruising
- flexible forefoot
- combination of nylon mesh and leather or suede uppers

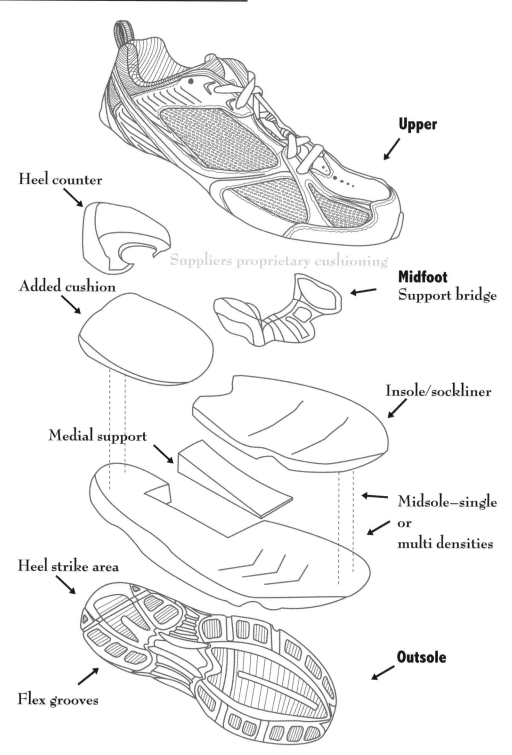

Upper

Heel counter

Suppliers proprietary cushioning

Added cushion

Midfoot
Support bridge

Insole/sockliner

Medial support

Midsole–single
or
multi densities

Heel strike area

Outsole

Flex grooves

Foot Characteristics for Each Shoe Type

1. Supportive Foot Characteristics

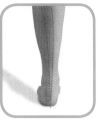 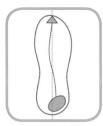 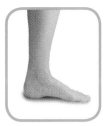 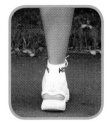

- feet and ankles roll inward (moderate—excessive, medially)
- low, flat arches
- knees and ankles move inward when bending or during heel strike
- if foot is not supported: knee pain, IT band, plantar fasciitis and shin splints

2. Cushioning Foot Characteristics

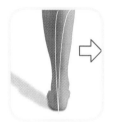 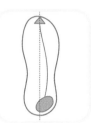 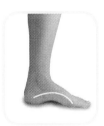 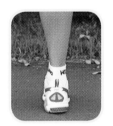

- knees and ankles roll to the outside (lateral)
- high and/or rigid arches
- underpronates
- if foot is not properly cushioned: stress fractures or pain on outside of shin or knee

3. Rugged Walk Foot Characteristics

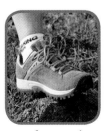 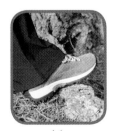 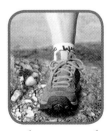

- foot strikes on an unstable environment, loose impediments
- walking on uneven ground
- moderate to severe up/downhill stride
- protection needed against rocks and roots on trail

How to Determine Your Foot Type

1. Wet Footprint

For this one, use a piece of paper and water. Wet your foot and make an imprint with your foot on the paper. Or, check out the floor as you exit the shower and see the foot imprint left behind. In either case look in the arch area; if you see a dry space between the heel and the ball of your foot, that would indicate you have a high, rigid arch, which means you have a neutral foot type or belong to the cushion category (yellow). If you see a portion of the area between the heel and the arch filled in, that would indicate your arch is lower and may in fact collapse, or flatten out entirely—which indicates you have a foot that moderately overpronates or belongs to the support category (blue). Both cushioning and support features are offered in rugged walking shoes (purple).

2. Feet Shoulder Width Apart

Bend at the knees and hold in that position. You will want to look at where your knees line up in respect to your big toe. Try to imagine a plumb line from the top of your knee to the top of your foot. If your knee is to the inside of the big toe, that would indicate that your feet have an inward/medial roll. You would want to look at the support category, depending on the degree of the roll. You can try shoes with varying degrees of medial support. The farther to the inside the knee comes the more support you will need. If the knee lines up more to the outside/lateral side of the big toe, that would indicate that your arch is more rigid and you would want to look at the cushion/neutral category. This is an easy way that you can get a good idea of how much support you will need.

3. Lunge Forward

Lunge forward and hold in that position. You will again be able to see where the knee is in comparison to the big toe (same as above). This will also work better if you have another person watching from the front. The person watching from the front should be looking at the knee position and also the arch and ankle. If the arch and ankle look very straight, then that would indicate more of a cushion category foot type. If the arch looks like it is starting to flatten and the ankle looks like it is starting to roll inward/medial, then that would indicate more of a support category foot type.

4. Old Shoes

If you have a pair of worn shoes, you can use them to read the wear pattern on the sole to get an idea of your foot type. Pick up your right shoe and turn the shoe upside down. You will most likely notice that there is some wear more toward the center of the heel or towards the left or lateral side of the shoe. This is normal wear. Almost all walkers make first contact with the ground at these points. If you look more towards the front of the shoe or the forefoot you will be able to get a really good idea what category you belong to. If you see wear on the far left/lateral side of the forefoot or more to the center, this would indicate that you belong to the cushion category. If you notice wear more to the right/medial side, that would indicate you belong to the support category. Also, the more the wear pattern is on the far right/medial side and towards the front of the shoes, the more medial support is needed in the shoe.

5. Have Someone Watch You Walk

If you are able, get a friend to watch you walk as normal as possible in bare or socked feet. They will want to look for some key characteristics such as ankle movement and knee movement. If you see the knee lining up with the top of the big toe and the ankle rolling in a straight position from heel to toe-off or movement to the outside or lateral side, then you need more cushioning. If you see the knee rolling inward/medial past the big toe and the ankle also rolling inward/medial, then this would indicate you need more support. If you notice the knee rolling excessively past the big toe and the ankle rolling inward in an excessive way, then this would be an indication to pick a shoe with more support that extends farther on the medial side. With this exercise, I suggest you walk towards and away from the person to give them a chance to see you from both directions.

Steps in Selecting the Best Shoe

Fitness walkers do not necessarily have to steer clear of running shoes. Shoes built for running will, in most cases, meet your needs very well. Walking shoes may not! If you find yourself looking at walking shoes, check that they have not actually been designed for moderate hiking or for those whose profession involves a lot of time on their feet. Look in the running shoe section and see what meets the needs of your gait. They will certainly be more numerous than walking shoes. Try several pairs; walk around in them. Evaluate them just as a walker would, in terms of your type of foot and your athletic needs. For your regular fitness walking and your power walking, a comfortable training shoe is what you need. If it happens to be called a running shoe, who cares?

If you are a race walker, your needs are more specific, especially if you are planning to compete. Genuine race walking shoes are quite rare; look for racing flats or lightweight trainers.

Racing flats are shoes made for walkers to race in. They sacrifice a lot of their cushioning to reduce weight. They are more flexible and accommodate a more dynamic racing stride. They are delicate, because they are not used in high mileage training. As a result, they provide a good "feel" for the road and a direct transfer of the athletes' power.

Lightweight trainers take advantage of advanced shoe technology to provide strength and stability without bulk. These days, you may find that your choice of lightweight trainers is more extensive than the selection of racing shoes. They are made for walkers who do not need the ample cushioning that traditional training shoes provide.

For these reasons, racing flats and lightweight trainers work well for race walkers. The low heel lends itself to our typical roll from heel to toe. The flexibility accommodates the final stage of our foot drive and our permanently cocked toes. An eminent coach once said that if you couldn't fold your race walking shoes up like a wallet, they weren't flexible enough! A slight exaggeration, but we take his point.

Your racing flats or lightweight trainers will last longer for race walkers because our impact is much less than walkers. A tip from experienced athletes: When you find a shoe you really like, buy as many pairs as you can afford. The nature of the industry is such that the exact same model may no longer be available when you go back for another pair a few months later.

Which Shoe Fits Your Style?

Good shoes are still the soundest investment you can make, and coupled with a sensible training schedule, essential in helping to prevent injury. So many shoes, so many configurations, with a little time and our expertise, the chances of finding one that works for you are excellent.

Trail and Off Road
Choose Rugged Walk
Characteristics

Footwear in this category is designed for the walker who requires athletic performance both on-off trail. Selected combinations of lightweight, breathable materials in the uppers provide support and comfort in a protective package. Cushioned midsole in multiple densities provide effective shock absorption.

Shoes will have a slightly more aggressive outsole design for a stable foot strike and durable traction over multi-surface terrain.

Protection is needed to ensure the foot lands on a stable cushioned platform. Any movement over uneven or loose ground can cause an ankle to turn or stone bruising underneath the foot. Best Last: Design is usually curved or semi-curved for responsive performance; midsole/outsole design allow for comfort, support and protection. Best Shoes: Stability shoes with firm midsoles, a wide landing base and control features, such as a strong, rigid heel counter, to keep the heel secure and reduce the degree of pronation as well as a posting on the medial side for added support and guidance.

Neutral
Choose Cushioning
Characteristics

Feet roll to outside, arches are high and/or rigid that usually do not pronate enough, and do not provide effective shock absorption, knees stay neutral or move outwards through foot strike. Shoe wears along the outside of the sole.

Injuries

Stress fractures, pain on outside of shin/knee. Best Last: Curved, slip-lasted shoe for low or moderate rearfoot stability. Best Shoes: Moderate rearfoot and pronation control. Lightweight cushioning shoes with a flexible forefoot and soft/firm midsole.

Normal-Excessive Pronator
Choose Stability
Characteristics

Normal-flat arch, lands on the outside of the heel and then rolls inward (pronates) to absorb shock. Semi-flexible arch that requires varied degrees of support. Knees roll in when bent. Best Last: Semi-curved/straight. Best Shoes: Supportive shoes with a degree of guidance features, such as moderate pronation support, strong heel counters and multidensity midsole. These provide extra cushioning and some degree of stability.

Tips for Shoe Buying

1. Spend Time

Walk in the shoe. Don't buy shoes because they worked well for someone else. Test them out.

2. Take Along Your Old Shoes, A Pair of Coolmax Socks and Your Orthotics

Our Walking Room staff can read your wear pattern, and it is important to be fitted with the Coolmax sock you will be walking in.

3. Tell Us...

About your walking history, goals, past injuries, the type of training you do and what has or hasn't worked for you in the past.

4. Walking Room Foot Exam

Whether you have a rigid or flexible foot, a low or high arch, or are flat-footed, they all make a difference as to what will best suit you.

5. Comfort

Pressure spots or loose fitting shoes will be susceptible to blisters. If your foot slides excessively, you will also lose energy on the push off.

6. A Snug Fit

Pull the laces so that you have a feeling of security without discomfort.

7. Selecting The Right "Last" (Footbed Construction)

All shoes are constructed over a wood or composite form called a "last." The three predominant shapes today are the straight, curved and semi-curved. If you have a curved foot and wear a straight shoe, you will feel pressure on the inside of your big toe, and you will tend to roll off the outside of the shoe.

8. The Selection Process

Select two or three models that work best for your foot function. Compare the fit of each and then stand and walk around in each shoe to feel how it performs. You will find your new shoes choose you.

Proper Shoe Selection

9. Walking In Cross Trainers or Aerobic Shoes?

Walking shoes are designed for a forward motion and cushion the impact specific to walking. Cross trainers and aerobic shoes are designed for more indoor use and have more lateral support and toe flexibility. If used as your walking shoes, you will risk injury over time.

10. When To Buy A New Pair

Often, a shoe's upper is still in great shape, but the cushioning and support has been lost. A test? Mark the date that you bought your shoes, and drop by the Walking Room after you have logged approximately 800 kilometers or 500 miles to compare your old shoes with a new pair. The key to keeping off the injury list is to replace your shoes once they begin to wear or break down.

Walking Gear and Accessories

Besides shoes, there's an almost endless variety of clothing and accessories that can make your walking more enjoyable. Below you will find a summary of basic clothing and accessory needs, what to look for and why. For a more detailed review of clothing needs related to weather, look in *Chapter 8, Walking and the Weather*.

Socks

Socks are important. After all, if your feet aren't comfortable, your walk won't be either. Socks have a range of thickness: thin, midweight and cushioning. They can be made with a single or double layer of fabric and all synthetics and wool that wick moisture away and help cushion your feet. Some socks have reflective lettering or markings on the ankle to help keep you visible after dark. Take along your shoes if you plan to buy socks, so you'll know exactly how they'll feel out on the road.

Outer Layer

A good jacket can take you from fall through to spring, when it's layered properly. Most importantly, you want a fabric that is windproof and breathable. Water resistant is also good. Vents along the back, zippered vents under the arms and adjustable sleeve cuffs allow you to control the amount of moving air flow you want on a particular day. Reflective strips are great for those winter walks when the daylight disappears long before your walk is over. Some jackets have a panel in the back that can drop down and cover your posterior, warding off the wind and rain, and a drawstring waist helps keep the wind out.

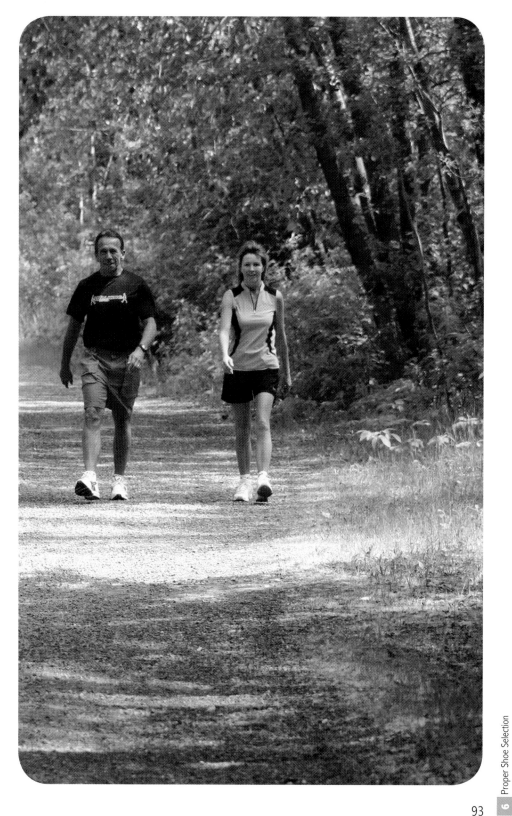

Zippered pockets are also helpful to hold keys and cell phone for an emergency phone call.

For all your walking gear, think fit, function and fashion. You want to look good, feel good and walk your best.

Base, Inner or Single Layer

Forget cotton. It absorbs moisture, which causes chafing on longer walks. Look for a synthetic fabric designed to wick moisture away from the body. A snug fit will allow the fabric to perform the wicking action. By doing so, you stay dry and cool in the heat and warmer in colder conditions.

Pants, Capris and Shorts

Look for fabric that wicks moisture away from the body. You want protection according to the seasons from the various elements like wind and rain.

Mid Layers

Look for fleece with the similar performance and functionality as the jacket. Typically, it should be a heavier weight fabric than your base layer. A multifunctional piece that can be worn on cold days or as the outerwear piece of a base layer. Look for a front zipper to allow for temperature control and small pockets to carry the essentials.

Underwear

Look for a technical fabric that will help carry the moisture from your skin to the next layer.

Women: A supportive bra is essential for comfort during your workout. Different features are needed to accommodate different shapes and sizes. Look for these items in high support bras:

- Encapsulated Cups
- Compression
- Adjustable Straps
- Hook and Eye Back Closure
- Non-Stretch Molded Cups

Men: For maximum protection during cold weather, especially in the wind, look for a boxer or brief with a wind panel.

Outer Layer

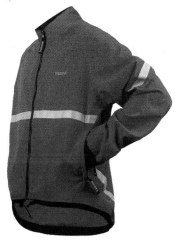

Inner Layer

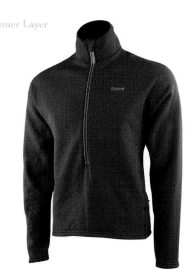

Capris

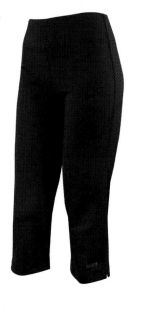

Pants

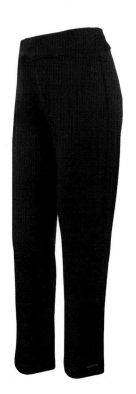

Socks

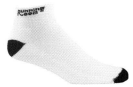

Socks

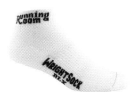

Proper Shoe Selection

6

Hats

A good percent of your body heat can be lost through the head, so a hat that covers the ears is needed in winter, and the face cover in very cold temperatures. Depending on the temperature, a band over the ears can do. In summer, a walking cap with a broad rim made of breathable fabric can protect from harmful UV rays and rain.

Mittens and Gloves

Your hands do very little work to generate heat during walking, so it is important to protect them from the cold. Look for windproof and wickable fabric. For colder conditions mittens are warmer than gloves.

Speed, Distance and Heart Rate

One of the biggest challenges for walkers has been to monitor the intensity of workouts, pace and distance. You will find lots of walking speedometers—odometers that claim they can tell you how far and how fast you are walking. However, many speedometers can be tricky to get calibrated for walking and rely on input of your stride length. They will always vary by 10% or more on distance, and therefore on speed. Technology now allows for the extremely simple and accurate speed and distance monitors to work right out of the box. Let's review what's available.

There are a number of methods of calculating walking speed, pace and distance. Some of these units use GPS like the Garmin® products. The GPS devices can be used for any outdoor sport, and most will download collected data to your computer. Every walker should have one. A single wrist unit uses GPS satellites to trace your outdoor workout. Displays speed, distance, pace, time and laps in large display. Chart your route as you walk, and it can point you back to start. Pace alerts and a virtual partner can pace your workout. You can download all data to a computer with the provided serial interface. It generally has free logbook software, or uses free online GPS Visualizer programs that come with the units. Many models are available with or without a heart rate monitor to help you make the most out of your training. Train in a certain heart rate zone to improve your fitness level or compare your pace and heart rate to past performance on the same workout.

Others use a highly accurate and sensitive accelerometer device that discreetly attaches to the shoe laces, Nike® and Polar®. These footpod devices are not like the basic pedometer we are most familiar with. They are highly accurate

Hats

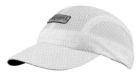

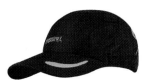

Underwear

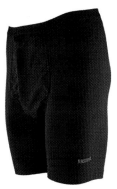

Mid Layers

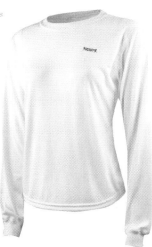

Underwear

Mittens and Gloves

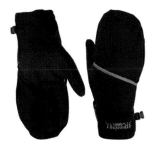

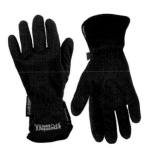

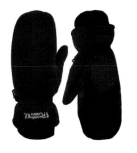

and they do not rely on the user to set stride length, etc. The Polar® Footpod accurately measures your walking speed/pace and distance. This essential piece of kit attaches to your laces and will be with you every step of the way. With the Nike® Sports Kit you put your sensor in your shoe, and you're ready to walk. The receiver connects to your iPod Nano, collecting workout data with every step. This pedometer sensor transmits data wirelessly to an iPod nano where you can view it and have it spoken to you over your music mix. It uses an accelerometer rather than GPS, so accuracy varies if your stride varies. It works indoors or outdoors.

What is GPS?

Global Positioning System (GPS) is the core technology behind many new products that track your training and wirelessly sends your data to your computer. Each walk is stored in its memory, so you can review and analyze the data to see how you've improved. Monitor your time, distance, pace and calories.

Originally developed in 1973 by the U.S. Department of Defense for military purposes, the NAVSTAR GPS network consists of 30 satellites orbiting the earth every 12 hours, and five ground stations that monitor the satellites' position in space and operational status. To determine your location and other data accurately, such as current and average speed, pace, directional heading and elevation, GPS devices use a receiver to acquire signals from at least four of these satellites to calculate the location within 10 meters. The device uses four simple data points (latitude, longitude, altitude and time) collected every few seconds.

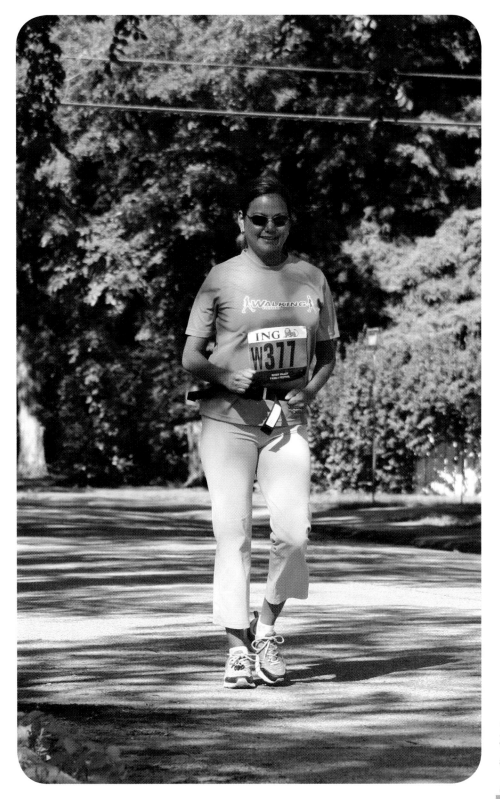

Walking Gear and Accessories Checklist Before the Event

Cap

A breathable, lightweight cap that will help keep you cool and keep the sun's damaging rays off you during the race is a good choice.

Water Bottle

Most good races will have adequate water along the course. If you're unsure of the frequency of the water stations, wear a torso pack to take your own water with you.

Shirt

Pick one that gives you both comfort with sun and wind protection.

Watches

A walker's watch is essential in gauging the intensity and duration of your workouts. It also gives the run/walk ratio. Be sure to get one that is waterproof and readable in the dark. Sometimes a watch, pedometer and heart rate monitor can all be found in the same device.

Gel Flask

Holds up to five gels and can be carried on a torso belt.

Shorts/Tights

There are some great technical fabrics that will keep you dry and chafe-free in a variety of conditions.

Pedometer

Pedometers are adjustable to your stride length to measure the distance walk/stroll. Some have a stopwatch.

Bodyglide/Slick Stick

Will keep you from chafing.

Race Number

Make sure you have it and make sure you pin it on the singlet or shirt that you will be wearing in the race. Take a few extra pins or race belt.

Duffel Bag

Keeps all your workout essentials organized in three separate compartments, shoes, dry clothes and wet clothes. Features a side pocket with a detachable key chain and waterproof pocket, adjustable strap and side reflectivity. 45L capacity.

Shoes

The best shoes to race in are the ones you trained in. Some folks like racing flats for shorter races, but with improved shoe technology making high-quality, lightweight trainers available, most opt for their training shoes.

Water Belt

Look for a light, snug fit around the waist so your bottle won't jiggle uncomfortably, even with an angled bottle. Some have pockets for keys, food and change, and they are insulated for your water to stay cold.

Socks

Choose a comfortable pair that you have used in training.

Gel

A must-have for long walks, giving you the extra energy to keep going.

Reflective Clothing and Acessories

Working out after dark or early in the morning? Make sure you can be seen. Reflective clothing and accessories add a measure of safety to your workout without adding a heavy layer. Reflective arm bands can be added to any walking outfit.

Heart Rate Monitor/GPS

Very complex monitors show heart rate, intensity, distance, repeats, GPS, memory and more. Monitors have become a tool for the modern walker.

Timing Chip

The new timing systems sometimes sell individual timing chips to racers. If you have one of these, be sure to take it along with you.

Your Training Program

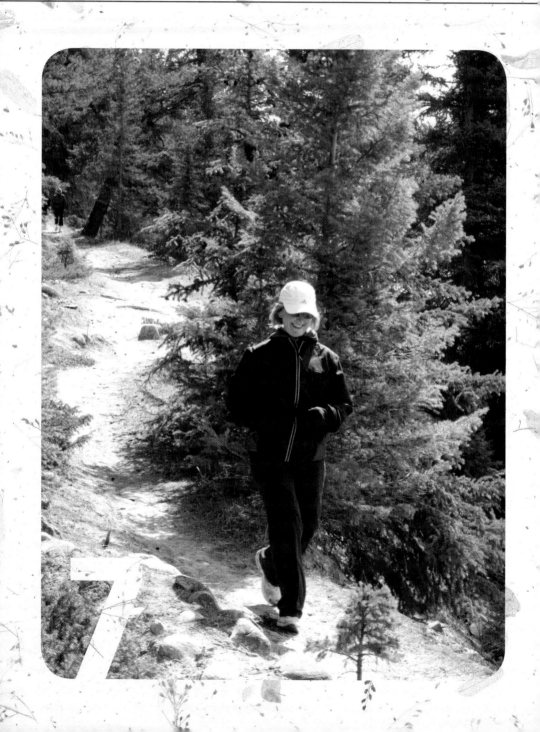

7

Getting Started

Monitoring Your Training Effort

Our bodies divide effort into three main physiological zones. First, there is a level of low-intensity activity when no real demands are being made on our system. As a result, little training is taking place. Second, there is a zone in that effective aerobic training is occurring. Third, there is a high-activity zone that is capable of great output sustainable only for a short time. In this zone, the body's defense mechanisms change the biochemistry of your energy production so that aerobic activity is actually prevented. The aerobic training effect, which walkers are seeking, lies in the middle zones.

One way is to use a heart rate monitor to train in the correct target zone. The heart rate monitor is your silent coach, which provides you with feedback on the correct level of intensity.

The zones are also divided by two physiological responses, which are easy for you to feel. These divisions correspond very closely to heart rates, which the monitors use in establishing the zones.

The transition from the first to the second zone is marked by the onset of sweat. When you sweat as a result of gentle exercise, your body's cooling mechanism is doing its job.

The transition from the second to the third zone is marked by the onset of labored breathing.

When your breathing slips out of a controlled, comfortable rhythm, you are not getting the oxygen you need. The old talk test also works well. If you can only gasp out three or four words at a time, you are entering the third zone and walking too fast. Slow down in order to return the effort to a sustainable and comfortable level. If you can talk non stop, you should pick up the pace a little.

Walk This Way

We have discussed how your fitness walking very likely takes one of four forms:

1. active walking for lifestyle improvement, additional recreational opportunities and the "I feel good" feeling of being an athlete

2. power walking and its increased effort improves the cardiovascular system and muscular skeletal strength

Your Training Program

7

3. athletic walking through fast-paced competitive walking and even race walking; fast walking is fun

4. race walking with its increased speed and possible competition—you compete with others to improve your own performance

The programs in this chapter can be done using any form of walking. Choose the program that most corresponds to your walking goals.

Why Training Works: Principles of Conditioning

Let's take a closer look at training, what it is and how and why it works.

Training works because of the human ability to adapt to stress. Incidentally, this ability applies to all kinds of stress, whether it's a physical load, a mental task or a crowded daily schedule. Within limits, we find stress challenging, invigorating and progressively easier to handle. As you improve your athletic goals, other areas of your life also improve.

There are two fundamental elements in this concept. The first is the stress itself. It has to be present for us to adapt and be stronger. The second is the periodic removal of the stress so adaptation can take place. Simply put, you get better at a physical activity when you are resting from it. Actually doing the activity makes you tired. As you rest, adaptation takes place so that you can do the activity better next time. Stress and rest is the principle of all training. Swimmers and track runners do intervals with high intensity followed by an interval of rest. Soccer players do wind sprints; all athletes include stress and rest in their training regimes

Training also works when you practice the specific activity. There are two elements in this concept. One, the more specific your goal, the more specific your preparation needs to be. If you want to be a better weight lifter, you can't rely on regular rounds of golf to help you out. Two, you have to "use it or lose it." If you stop your preparation, or reduce the level of stress below what is necessary for adaptation, then de-training, the opposite of training, occurs.

So we have two concepts with two elements each. These four elements provide us with four fundamental principles of training: They are progressive loading, adaptation, specificity and reversibility. An understanding of these simple principles and the way in which you build them into your own training will yield you the best results.

These principles will guide the structure of your training and gear your goals to your success. You may have to change your way of looking at your training a little bit.

Principles of Training

Progressive Loading

The physiological system strengthens only when it is regularly exposed to loads greater than those previously encountered. Continue to challenge yourself for improvement.

Adaptation

The physiological system strengthens during recovery from the training loads. Rest allows for recovery as you become stronger.

Specificity

Training loads must match the requirement of the activity in which enhanced performance is sought. To walk faster, you must walk faster. To walk longer, you must walk longer.

Reversibility

The physiological system will revert to previous levels if training loads are increased. Use it or you will lose it.

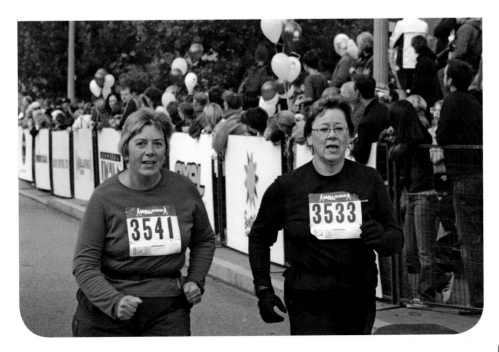

Ten-Week Conditioning Programs

In this section we will introduce three levels of the conditioning programs: introductory, intermediate and advance programs. These programs are intended to take the beginner walker and introduce them to a structured walking program in preparation for more advanced training programs that follow in the book (see pages 108 and 115).

1. Introductory Program
Goals

Change lifestyle with regular training.
Increase cardiovascular fitness and strength by comfortably completing three training sessions per week.
Learn fundamental fitness concepts through personal experience.
Start with a steady continuous walk for 20 to 30 minutes. Don't stop unless you really have to. But slow down any time that you find yourself short of breath.

Once you can walk steadily for 30 minutes without a break, you can begin the intermediate schedule. We increase the effort by introducing periods of quicker walking. This pattern of alternating periods of greater effort to provide a training load with periods of reduced effort to provide a rest and recovery is the basic structure of interval training, which all competitive athletes use. It will work for you, too.

To increase the effort, you just stride out, or use your arms more. At this point, you will pretty much be power walking. You can get the same effort by walking up a hill.

The following schedule should be done at least three times per week for best results. We have included two selections for each week. The first one is a pleasant longer walk and the second one is structured to capitalize on the principles of interval training.

In the longer walk, keep the pace as gentle as you need with the aim of maintaining it for the duration of the session. However, if you do need a recovery break, take it.

Do both sessions each week. The third session is a choice of either of the other two. In our example program, we have repeated a more structured workout, which incorporates the walk stroll intervals. You are welcome to repeat the continuous longer walks as an option. Exception: Weeks 4 and 9 are adaptation weeks. The third session is to repeat the gentle walk.

A proper warm-up and cooldown should be part of each session. These activities are not built into the session time listed in the program. For best effect, space the sessions throughout the week. Take at least two days between the two sessions, which are the same.

Words of Wisdom about a Training Program

1. This program starts conservatively, and builds in intensity and duration.

2. Consistency of training is very important. Once you reach the halfway mark of this program, you may find it difficult to maintain the progression unless you train three times per week. But by then you will be motivated and enjoy walking.

3. Your body needs time to adapt to increased training. The normal recovery days should do this for you. But notice that the volume actually drops in Weeks 4 and 9. This is done to allow the necessary adaptation to the previous weeks. Stress and rest will show in many forms in your training.

4. If you miss training time, consider it recovery. Start again at a level you can handle, even if it means dropping back a level. If you have been ill, we recommend doing so; even if you feel better, your body may take a little longer to completely recover.

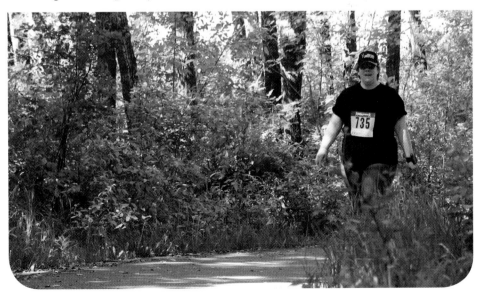

Throughout the program, walk refers to your preferred form of fitness walking. The assumption is that it will be brisk. For your recovery, we use the word "stroll," indicating a gentle relaxed normal walk.

10-Week Conditioning Program—Introductory

Week	Walks Per Week	Daily Session	Description	Walking Time	Session Time
1	3	a	Walk 1 minute, stroll 2 minutes. Do 6 sets, then add another 1 minute walk to finish	7	19
		b	Walk gently for 30 minutes	30	
		c	Walk 1 minute, stroll 2 minutes. Do 6 sets, then add another 1 minute walk to finish	7	19
2	3	a	Walk 1 minutes, stroll 1 minute. Do 10 sets	10	20
		b	Walk gently for 30 minutes	30	
		c	Walk 1 minutes, stroll 1 minute. Do 10 sets	10	20
3	3	a	Walk 2 minutes, stroll 1 minute. Do 6 sets, then add another 2 minute walk to finish	14	20
		b	Walk gently for 35 minutes	35	
		c	Walk 2 minutes, stroll 1 minute. Do 6 sets, then add another 2 minute walk to finish	14	20

Adaptation Week - Volume drops in Week 4

Week	Walks Per Week	Daily Session	Description	Walking Time	Session Time
4	3	a	Walk 3 minutes, stroll 1 minute. Do 5 sets	15	20
		b	Walk gently for 30 minutes. Compare feeling with Week 1	30	
		c	Walk 3 minutes, stroll 1 minute. Do 5 sets	15	20
5	3	a	Walk 4 minutes, stroll 2 minutes. Do 4 sets	16	24
		b	Walk gently for 40 minutes	40	
		c	Walk 4 minutes, stroll 2 minutes. Do 4 sets	16	24
6	3	a	Walk 5 minutes, stroll 2 minutes. Do 3 sets	15	21
		b	Walk gently for 40 minutes	40	
		c	Walk 5 minutes, stroll 2 minutes. Do 3 sets	15	21
7	3	a	Walk 4 minutes, stroll 1 minute. Do 5 sets	20	25
		b	Walk gently for 50 minutes	50	
		c	Walk 4 minutes, stroll 1 minute. Do 5 sets	20	25
8	3	a	Walk 3 minutes, stroll 1 minute. Do 6 sets	18	24
		b	Walk gently for 55 minutes	55	
		c	Walk 3 minutes, stroll 1 minute. Do 6 sets	18	24

Adaptation Week - Volume drops in Week 9

Week	Walks Per Week	Daily Session	Description	Walking Time	Session Time
9	3	a	Walk 2 minutes, stroll 1 minute. Do 10 sets	20	30
		b	Walk gently for 40 minutes. Compare feeling with Week 5	40	
		c	Walk 2 minutes, stroll 1 minute. Do 10 sets	20	30
10	3	a	Walk 5 minutes, stroll 1 minute. Do 5 sets	25	30
		b	Walk gently for 60 minutes	60	
		c	Walk 5 minutes, stroll 1 minute. Do 5 sets	25	30

2. Intermediate Program

+ To use the fitness gained in the introductory period in structured training sessions.

+ To improve personal achievement as a result of the lifestyle change that regular training requires.

When you can walk gently for one hour and can do the interval sessions in the introductory program with confidence, you are ready for the intermediate program. You will have noticed an improvement in your capabilities. Each session may still have its challenges; some will feel better than others. But you are able to look back a few weeks and realize just how far you have come and how much stronger you have become.

The improvement in fitness is not just in your aerobic system, which is made up of your heart, lungs and circulation. The time you have been spending on your feet will have strengthened your muscles and skeleton.

Just as importantly, your training will have also strengthened your connective tissue, such as tendons and ligaments that link the body's structures together. Connective tissue is very often the site of the overuse injuries typical of endurance activity.

Best of all, the introductory goal of changing your lifestyle has been accomplished. You discover your training is now part of your lifestyle; you cannot image a day without training. The people you live with start to encourage you to train because they see the psychological improvements.

In this stage of the program, we continue to list three sessions per week. Your increased fitness and strength means that you may well feel like training more often. Take normal commonsense precautions, such as having good shoes, regularly stretching and doing proper warm-ups. You can add one or two moderate, gentle walks on other days without undue fear of injury. You can continue with the other activities you enjoy. If you begin to feel the accumulation of fatigue from one day to the other, take a day or two of rest. In your walking program, the three sessions below are the important ones.

If you are involved in power walking or race walking, you will certainly spend time on technique. This skill training can be done as part of a warm-up during a longer walk or as a specific session all to itself.

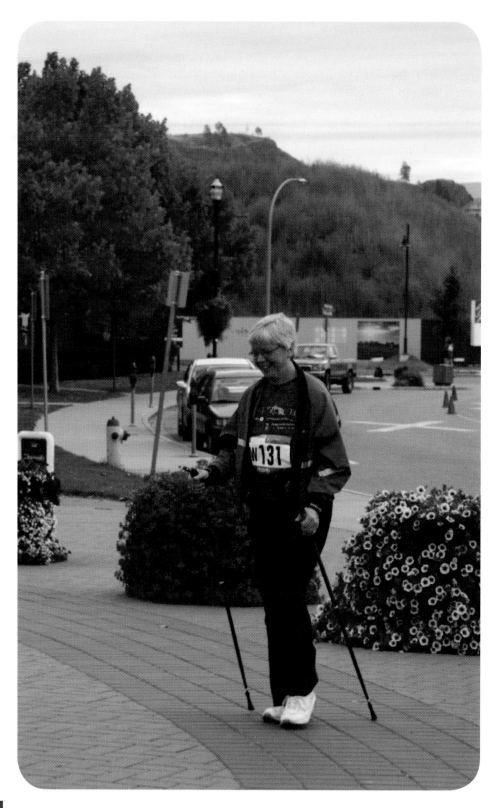

How We Introduce Increased Effort

Interval Training

You will notice that the structured workouts in this stage of the program involve periods of effort over a comparatively short distance followed by a period of recovery. Most of us use the generic term "interval training" to describe this pattern. We will look at interval training in more detail later, but here are the basic terms you will hear used.

We call these periods of effort, repetitions or sometimes repeats or reps, to use jargon. Each repetition is followed by a recovery. Reps are often grouped into sets. Sets are separated from each other by a slightly longer recovery called a set break. A good guide for a set break is that you do not start a set until you can feel like you can complete the full set. As you improve in fitness, you will find that this point is likely to be in the region of two or three minutes, a great time for a drink of water.

Many athletes also use the word "interval" in the same sense as repetition. Interval means the recovery between repetitions, but time has completely reversed the usage and many athletes interchange the words interval and repetition.

Speed Play

In the intermediate program, we use a structure of interval training that athletes often call fartlek, the Swedish word for speed play. Fartlek is less precise than a traditional interval workout where repetitions and recoveries are designed and strictly measured or timed. During speed play you don't stop during a set. You just slow down to a stroll and continue to your next starting point at a pace comfortable for you at the time. The repetitions are generally quite short, and you don't need to time them.

The control lies very much in your hands. Speed play sessions are a great way to escape any "blahs" you may be feeling from training or life in general. The only expectations you should have—finish feeling exhilarated. You should feel strong and enthusiastic, given your control of the intensity and duration of the interval. These sessions add spark and a change to your walking routine.

A traditional speed workout is done on a regular 400 meter track, with periods of effort along each straight and recovery periods around each bend. But a speed workout can be done anywhere.

Speed play can even be incorporated into a longer walk. You pick an upcoming landmark, such as a parked car, a lamppost or a tree, for your starting point and another as your finish. Or you simply glance at your watch and use a period of time for your effort and recovery. On the program sheet, we suggest an easy conversion. For each 100 meters, calculate approximately 45–60 seconds. If you are race walking and you find yourself closer to 30 seconds with your technique and form intact, you may very well be a champion walker.

Learning Your Technique

The speed play sessions are especially appropriate in the early stages of a walking program because of the way we learn new skills. Our brains need some time to get used to the new action. As our coordination improves, we hold our form longer.

This is part of your training. Our nervous system gets fatigued in a way physiologists still don't fully understand. We know that a brief rest from a new action allows us to try the action again. We know that this pattern of brief rehearsal and recovery periods is more effective than continuing under fatigue. We also know that rehearsing an action past the point of fatigue simply means that we are practicing poor form.

Speed Play of the Intermediate Walking Program

We have listed two speed play sessions per week. Your other session is a long walk.

The speed play sessions can be done at every level of fitness walking; it's your choice. You simply walk faster at a brisk pace for the period of effort and stroll for the recovery. Try to keep your recovery between repetitions no more than twice as long as the period of effort. I have listed set breaks at two to three minutes. If you need more, take them. If you can't see yourself completing the next set under control while maintaining your form, increase your stroll time until you can.

The long walk is to continue building your base. In a long walk, the time you spend walking is much more important than your speed or intensity. For active walking and power walking, set off at a pace you know you can maintain for 10 minutes. Take a one-minute stroll, or rest if you need it, and set off again for another 10 minutes. You are now part of my 10 and 1 system, which alternates 10 minutes of effort with one minute of recovery. The system has taken thousands of people to their goals of increased fitness or competitive success. These are commonly called 10 and 1's.

If you are race walking, I have one more consideration. As you begin to acquire the skill your form improves, but we cannot expect you to maintain it for 10 minutes at a time. Start your 10 minutes with a comfortable race walk and maintain it as long as it feels comfortable. There will likely come a point where you feel that you have lost your coordination. A beginner will often find the brisk walking for one minute and strolling for one minute a challenge. Your next session would be brisk walking for two minutes and strolling for one minute. From here, just continue to add the additional one minute of brisk walking. You will quite quickly progress to the point where you can continue the race walk for the entire 10 minutes.

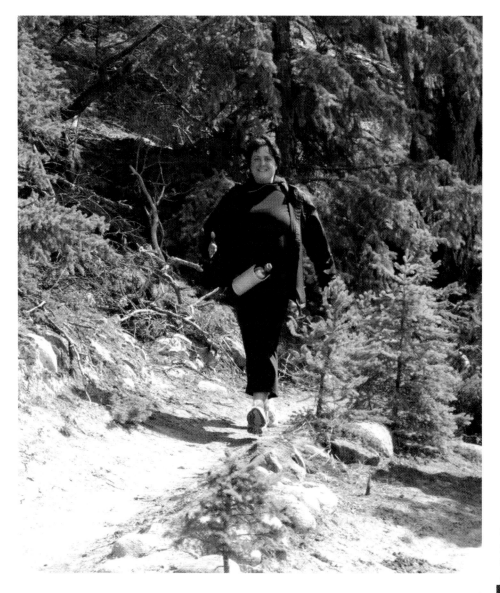

Ten-Week Intermediate Walking Program

Throughout the program, the word "walk" refers to your preferred form of fitness walking. The assumption is that it will be brisk. For your recovery, we use the word "stroll," indicating a gentle relaxed walk with friends.

A warm-up and cooldown is assumed to be part of every session

Your speed play sessions [(a) and (c), see chart] can be done for distance or time. Do them for distance if you are on a regular track or if you are confident that the measurement is accurate. Do them for a specific time if you do not know the distance or if you are including the session in a longer walk. Approximations are fine; speed play does not require precise measurements.

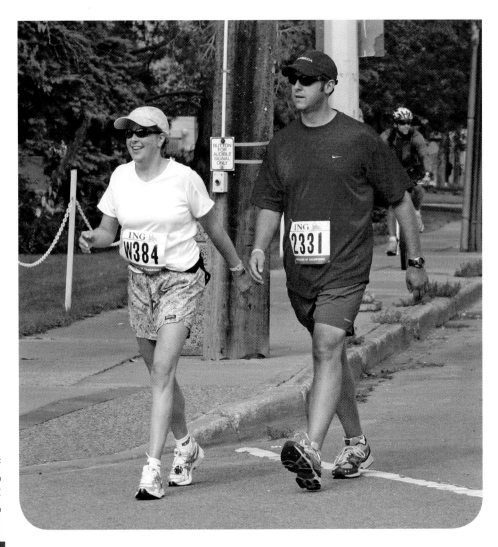

10-Week Conditioning Program—Intermediate

Week	Walks Per Week	Daily Session	Description	Workout
1	3	a	2 sets of 4 x 100 m fast walk, set break of 2–3 minutes stroll	Interval
		b	Long walk of 60 minutes	Steady Walk
		c	2 sets of 4 x 100 m fast walk, set break of 2–3 minutes stroll	Interval
2	3	a	3 sets of 3 x 100 m fast walk, set break of 2–3 minutes stroll	Interval
		b	Long walk of 60 minutes	Steady Walk
		c	3 sets of 3 x 100 m fast walk, set break of 2–3 minutes stroll	Interval
3	3	a	2 sets of 4 x 150 m fast walk, set break of 2–3 minutes stroll	Interval
		b	Long walk of 60 minutes	Steady Walk
		c	2 sets of 4 x 150 m fast walk, set break of 2–3 minutes stroll	Interval

Adaptation Week - Volume drops in Week 4

Week	Walks Per Week	Daily Session	Description	Workout
4	3	a	2 sets of 4 x 100 m fast walk, set break of 2–3 minutes stroll	Interval
		b	Long walk of 50 minutes	Steady Walk
		c	2 sets of 4 x 100 m fast walk, set break of 2–3 minutes stroll	Interval
5	3	a	3 sets of 3 x 150 m fast walk, set break of 2–3 minutes stroll	Interval
		b	Long walk of 65 minutes	Steady Walk
		c	3 sets of 3 x 150 m fast walk, set break of 2–3 minutes stroll	Interval
6	3	a	1 set or 4 x 100 m, 1 set of 3 x 150 m, 1 set of 2 x 200 m fast walk, set break of 2–3 minutes stroll	Interval
		b	Long walk of 65 minutes	Steady Walk
		c	1 set of 4 x 100 m, 1 set of 3 x 150 m, 1 set of 2 x 200 m fast walk, set break of 2–3 minutes stroll	Interval
7	3	a	1 set of 4 x 150 m, 1 set of 3 x 200 m fast walk, set break of 2–3 minutes stroll	Interval
		b	Long walk of 70 minutes	Steady Walk
		c	1 set of 4 x 150 m, 1 set of 3 x 200 m fast walk, set break of 2–3 minutes stroll	Interval
8	3	a	1 set of 8 x 100 m	Interval
		b	Long walk of 70 minutes	Steady Walk
		c	3 sets of 4 x 150 m, fast walk, set break of 2–3 minutes stroll	Interval

Adaptation Week - Volume drops in Week 9

Week	Walks Per Week	Daily Session	Description	Workout
9	3	a	3 sets of 3 x 150 m, fast walk, set break of 2–3 minutes stroll	Interval
		b	Long walk of 55 minutes	Steady Walk
		c	3 sets of 3 x 150 m, fast walk, set break of 2–3 minutes stroll	Interval
10	3	a	1 set of 3 x 150 m, 1 set of 4 x 200 m, 1 set of 4 x 100 m fast walk, set break of 2–3 minutes stroll	Interval
		b	Long walk of 75 minutes	Steady Walk
		c	3 sets of 4 x 200 m, stroll of 2–3 minutes	Interval

Ten-Week Advanced Training Program

Goal

+ Increase training density by comfortably completing more training sessions in a week, to a maximum of five.

+ Become familiar with the variables of interval training.

Introducing Hill Training

You are now at the point where a repertoire of training options opens to you. Your training need never be boring, your horizons are wide and your choices are many. In this section, we'll introduce you to some of those options and the terminology you will need to perform and speak like an athlete. We also look at interval and hill training in more detail.

Each session is designed around the principles of training. Understanding what your workout is intended to achieve is much more important than its details.

In the earlier stages of training, I supply exact workouts as a guide so you can understand the principles working for you and gain an understanding of how your body responds. At your stage of training now there is no magic in the exact number of kilometers walked or exact number of hills or speed intervals walked. Progressive loading, adaptation, specificity and reversibility—it's like a recipe for your favorite dish or those design plans for your new house. Plan for success and you will succeed. Without a plan you risk discouragement or even injury.

Two Recovery Days

This structure is perfectly adequate for most purposes. If you become involved in a program of competition where some events or races are more important to you than others and some times of the year are busier than others, you will find yourself wanting to adapt the structure. You will want to peak for that big races at other times. This is known as periodization, the periods of training and recovery to meet specific goals. There are a number of resources available if you wish to learn more.

Long and Moderate Walks

The long walk should be the longest session of the week. Let's start it at about 55 minutes. Any shorter and you won't consider it long enough with your new level of fitness. Unless you are planning on walking a marathon or getting ready for a hiking holiday, your long walk need not extend past the 75 minutes you did at the end of the introductory program.

We're not going to schedule the moderate walks for you; just get moving and enjoy them. Make walking part of your daily activities like brushing your teeth.

Interval Training

In the introductory and intermediate programs, we have become familiar with the concept of interval training, its vocabulary and its structure. But all we have done up to now is scratch the surface of its potential as a training vehicle. We started with some gentle repetitions and progressed into speed play. In the advanced program, we look closely at interval training. It does not take long to realize that we have at our disposal a training resource limited only by our imagination.

We have certainly figured out that interval training can be challenging. After some of your speed play session you ended up both pleasantly tired and elated. Other sessions may not have felt so good. Whether you struggled or triumphed, you sure did the session. You may like the discipline interval training imposes, or hate its relentless structure. Either way, you know that it's making you a stronger and better athlete.

As you enter the advanced program, you need to meet a new training standard. Doing so will help you to understand the principles behind interval training. As we progress, we find ourselves constantly checking back in our training logs to see what our log told us following previous sessions. We use this information to move our present training along. Regular competitors use specific planning for their upcoming races.

Think of a basic interval workout you have done in relative comfort. Let's take the last workout of the intermediate program as an example: three sets of four by 200 meters, set breaks of two to three minutes.

The workout has four elements: the length of the effort (200 meters), the number of repetitions (three sets of four), your speed as you did them and the amount of recovery time you take between each repetition and each set.

When building a program we need to consider recovery time, the number of repetitions, the length of the session and the intensity or speed of the session.

Starting from our basic workout, you are achieving a progression when the 200s can be done with less recovery than previously. If you started at a 2:1 recovery to effort ratio and you are able to reduce the ration to five minutes of effort to one

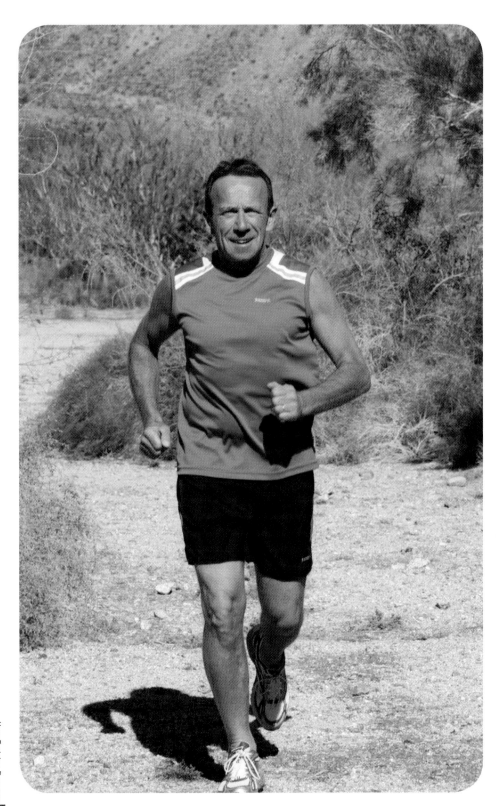

minute of recovery, you are significantly fitter than before. At that point, you can increase the amount of repetitions done from three to five as an example. When you've achieved that progression, you can increase the length of each repetition, which further increases the total distance you cover at a rhythm and form you can comfortably handle.

The speed of the effort is the last thing to be increased. Don't attempt to consciously increase your speed until you have achieved considerable progress on your rhythm and form.

There will be a natural improvement in speed as your brain, your muscles and your fitness respond to the training. Remember, we don't need blazing speed in walking, even in race walking. We just need to keep our personal rhythm and form solid for the distance we want to cover. Through training we maintain our form even as we tire.

As your program progresses, your total distance will be increasing significantly, and so will the training effort. Go back through the plan a second time if you like—reduce the recovery time, or do another set, or move up to even longer repetitions. But you and you alone decide when you are ready for the challenge. The real test is to keep more or less the same rhythm and maintain good technique and form.

Hill Training

Hills are speed work in disguise and a wonderful way to add some resistance to your training. When you overcome resistance, your muscles get stronger and the intensity of your training increases. Walkers have used hills for decades as a way to increase endurance, strength and speed.

You need only a long gentle slope, approximately an 8–10% grade at most. The hill should be a resistance, not an obstacle. You should be able to maintain your normal rhythm and technique as you start up the hill and maintain it, with a little more effort, as you get to the top.

Hills overload our cardiovascular system and shift our weight forward on our feet much like we do when walking faster. The up hill stress sessions improve our strength and form. We rest, and recovery is on the down hill.

If you live in the flatlands, you may have to resort to a bridge or underpass somewhere. The Canadian city Winnipeg converted an old garbage dump into a park that positively towers over the surrounding prairie plains The dubious honor of the only hill in town belongs to the road up to the top of the dump. If you are really stuck for a hill, you might have to find a tall building with friendly security guards and use the stairs. If you live in northern latitudes, stairs also come in useful in the cold dark days of winter. Covered parking ramps also offer an alternative, but check with the owners. These ramps are often quiet in the evenings and well lit.

Five Guidelines for Your Advanced Program

At this point in your training, there is such a wide horizon available to you and so many workout options that no general training schedule can cover all the possibilities. Your understanding of the principles of training and the way in which your body responds to training are now your greatest assets.

First and foremost, the right choice is the one that feels good for you. Rely on the keen sense of your own abilities that you develop as you progress.

Like all athletes, you are making selections from a world of opportunity opening up at your feet. You can enjoy the choices you now have, but you need not feel overwhelmed by them.

Re-read the section on the principles of conditioning (page 104) any time you feel that you are losing focus or you are not sure of what kind of training to do. In the advanced program, the following five guidelines may also help with some of the most common difficulties athletes encounter.

1. To achieve the best training effect, work with your body's basic physiology, not against it.

Your body has defense mechanisms that are designed to protect you. Trying to push through these defense mechanisms is actually an obstacle to the training effect you are trying to achieve.

As a competitive athlete, you will learn how to work at higher levels of intensity. The secret is to work very hard using a combination of rest and recovery.

Athletes understand that high intensity training or racing and base training are physiologically incompatible. Training on a rest day is counterproductive.

2. The body responds to training best when it has adequate recovery.

Rest is a part of all training. The more you advance, the more important rest and recovery become.

3. The body responds to training in a series of waves, in which training loads are followed by periods of adaptation to the loads.

On a graph, the progression of improvement follows a consistent pattern, but it is not a straight line. It is a series of waves undulating upwards. Each crest is followed by a trough, but each trough and each crest is higher than the previous one.

This graph demonstrates that it is quite normal for you to feel better on some days than on others during your workout. Evaluate your progress in the long term. Ask yourself if your workout is actually one that was beyond your capabilities a couple of months ago.

There is about one month of adaptation between applying a training load and feeling the positive effect of that training. Your achievements today are as the result of the training you did several weeks or months ago.

4. Train to your weakness.

By the time you have reached the advanced program, you will know your training strengths and weaknesses. You either look forward to interval sessions, or dread them. You may love the longer walks, or they may bore you to tears. You may never dream of missing a weight room session, or you may find yourself very busy every weight training day.

These preferences are completely understandable. There is a natural tendency to train to your strengths, to do the training you like the most. You are not alone. We all do this.

In the advanced programs for the 10K, half marathon and marathon training schedules all the components of training—tempo runs, fartlek workouts, hill work and speed work—that apply to your chosen activity contribute to your success. More importantly, neglecting a component will leave a gap in your program when you actually need these workouts the most.

Develop strategies to ensure that your least favorite workouts are still included:

+ Training with other people is almost guaranteed to relieve the stress. The group gives you the lift you need to do the workout.

+ Long, gentle warm-ups get you in the mood to finish a workout that you weren't too keen on starting. I use the 10-minute test on days when I do not feel like doing an interval session. I give myself permission to cut the session off after 10 minutes of easy walking if I am still tired. Invariably, I continue once I discover I was only mentally tired not physically tired.

+ If you are the structured type, structuring your workout completely often leaves you no choice but to get it done.

+ If your approach is a little less formal, deciding to do a little bit less than the ideal workout is still better than avoiding it entirely.

5. The details of a workout don't matter. The physiological purpose of the workout matters a lot.

Training schedules look so convenient. The schedule of elite athletes, a colleague you admire or a rival you want to beat looks so appealing. The fact is there is nothing magic about a certain mileage, a certain number of repetitions or a certain speed. Our programs are examples presented with clarity.

Good coaches will watch for each athlete's response to particular training loads and then adapt the session accordingly. For example, a workout of 10 hills of 250 meters can be adapted in many ways. If an athlete is doing well, he or she can do all 10. Another might run into trouble halfway though. That athlete can rest for one repetition and then join back in. Doing nine reps well is better than doing five well and then struggling through five, just because the workout sheet says to do 10. The key is to run all the hills with good strong form. Why practice poor form!

Others may respond better by stopping each hill at 200 meters. The extra rest may allow them to maintain their best rhythm and form. This is more effective for their training than trudging up the remaining 50 meters with poor rhythm and form.

Keep your training quantity, time and distance at an amount that challenges you when you are doing it, but allows for complete recover after 48 hours of rest.

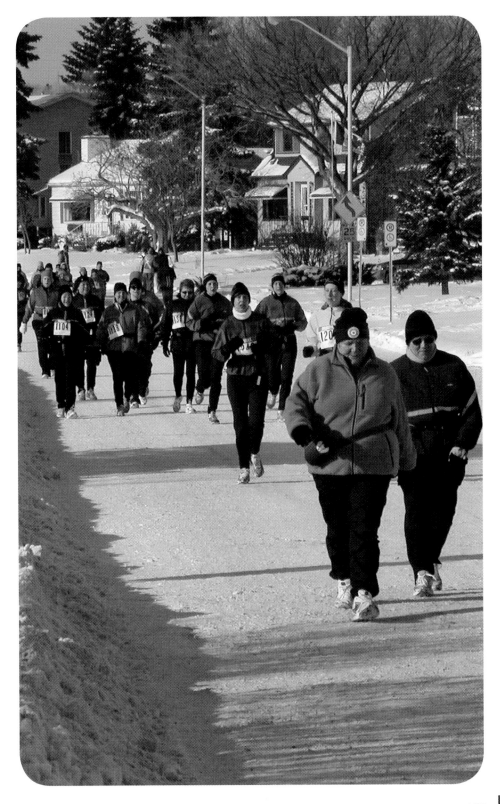

Three Levels of Walking
More About Active Walking

Walking is one of our most natural motions. But we can make some suggestions as a checklist and a base from which you can progress efficiently.

Good posture is the core of walking technique and form. Posture is the result of muscles working in the way in which nature intended. Keep your head up: look in front of you, not down. Relax your shoulders and neck muscles. Walk tall by gently contracting the stomach muscles and the gluteus, the cheeks of your butt. Tilt the pelvis slightly, tucking it under your body and allowing the hips to move the legs forward more easily and with improved alignment.

These basic movements are part of good walking technique or form. In an exercise program, technique is rarely something you change just by thinking about it. It is a longer process. The muscles strengthen in order to do a movement that is slightly different than the one they have been used to for years. Your brain needs to learn a slightly different movement, which takes time. Compare the learning process to any other skill. Any new movements feel awkward at first.

We have defined active walking as normal walking done as a lifestyle choice. Our walking has a clear purpose. Here's how the purpose is translated into action.

+ Pick up the pace just a little. This boosts the intensity of your walking. You will start to sweat, a sure sign that your heart rate is moving up into the aerobic training zone. You may notice a slightly longer stride as you pick up the speed. That's fine, but don't seek additional stride length just for the sake of it. Instead, listen to your feet. Actually count the rhythm of your strides and notice that the rhythm becomes quicker. This additional stride frequency, or turnover, are keys to increasing your fitness.

+ Notice your arm swing. With your more purposeful stride, you'll need an arm swing to match. When you are strolling, your arms are really just along for the ride and to provide a little balance. They do the same when you pick up the pace. Don't let people tell you that your arms drive you forward. They don't, but they are a useful reminder of what your legs are doing. When you start moving even faster, you will find yourself using your arms to coax some extra drive out of your legs. Consider your arm swing as a metronome to maintain your rhythm.

More about Power Walking

Power walking is actually not a specific technique. Power walking is a form of walking that is designed to add effort, and therefore fitness benefits, to active walking. Power walking involves deliberately accentuated actions of the arms and legs. When you power walk, you have set out to work harder than you do during a pleasant or long walk home from work.

Some power walkers add other arm movements as they walk: overhead extensions or lateral raises. If you are comfortable, add these elements of an aerobics workout to your walking.

I do not recommend the use of weights while power walking. Strength training is more effective when done in separate sessions. Aerobic training done with natural movements significantly reduces the risk of injury. Walking is almost injury-free anyway; let's keep it that way. If you want to increase the aerobic load, just walk faster.

Long-arm Power Walking

To start power walking, you can simply increase the intensity of your active walking one more level. Your arms will swing from the shoulders like a military quick march. You will breathe more heavily, and at times may even approach the labored breathing level that marks the beginning of your departure from the aerobic training zone. At this point, it is best for you to slow down.

With the long arm swing, your stride will tend to be longer too. You will certainly feel that the stride is more powerful. You may hear a louder foot plant. The stride rate may actually slow down because on each stride you need time to haul yourself up and over your foot, which is extended out in front of you.

Long-arm power walking may be the effort you were looking for as a fitness activity. There is nothing at all wrong with long-arm power walking. You will increase the intensity and you will engage more muscle groups to work more dynamically. It is one of your options.

Short-arm Power Walking

A small adjustment to your basic long-arm power walk will add another dimension to the activity. Bend your arms at the elbow and hold them as if you were running. Think of a pendulum. Hold the string at the end and the pendulum swings at a certain rate. Grab the string halfway down and the pendulum swings at a quicker rate. A shorter lever moves faster.

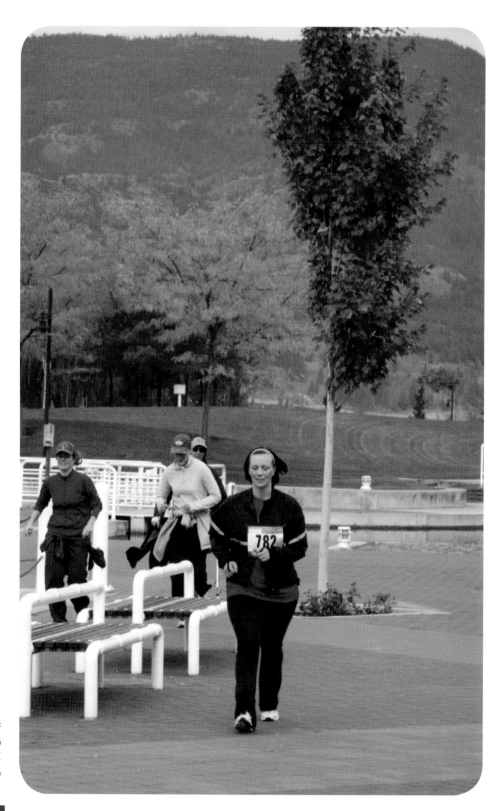

Bending your arms has the same effect. You can move your bent arm more quickly than your fully extended one. Many power walkers do this naturally. At this point, you may actually be race walking.

More about Athletic Walking

Athletic walking includes fast-paced walking, competitive walking and race walking. For our purposes here, I will address the fastest form of walking—race walking. Race pace walking is the name given to the fastest kind of walking there is. Because it is the form of walking used in competition, race walking is defined very specifically. You don't have to race to race walk. You can simply use the fast and efficient action to increase the effects of your walking program dramatically.

Everything in race walking is designed for speed. You may not wish to participate in a race, but you will be able to walk faster than you ever thought possible.

More about Race Walking

There are two principal elements to the definition of race walking. First, there must be the appearance of unbroken contact with the ground. Second, the supporting leg must be straight when the foot hits the ground. Then, it must stay straight until it is directly under the body.

Race walkers call infringing these rules lifting and creeping respectively. In race walking races there are judges to make sure the rules are followed.

If you're race walking for fitness, or walking in a half or even full marathon, you don't have to worry about judges. You may even find that some of the actions of race walking are difficult for you. You'll find that working on your technique makes your walking look and feel better. If you're in the vast majority, you will improve with practice and experience. In the meantime, just walk.

If you decide you want to go in a judged race at some stage, you'll need to make sure your technique is okay. You would do the same if you entered a volleyball tournament.

The actual definition is in the *Handbook of the International Amateur Athletic Federation* (IAAF). It's Rule 230.1 in the 2000/01 handbook. Frankly, the wording is awkward, but you can see what the two basic elements are. Here goes:

IAAF Rule 230.1 (2000–2001 edition)

"Race walking is a progression of steps so taken that the walker makes contact with the ground so that no visible (to the human eye) loss of contact occurs. The advancing leg shall be straightened (i.e., not bent at the knee) from the moment of first contact with the ground until the vertical upright position."

The Four Easy Steps and One Tricky One!

You can make a transition from normal walking to race walking in four easy stages and one tricky one! You can do this as a warm-up for each session if you like. You can also do it any time you feel your technique or your coordination starting to break down as it often will in the early stages. When this happens, don't hesitate to go back to a normal walk and start the transition again. You're just giving yourself a brief rest!

Step One

While walking normally, bend your elbow to 90 degrees. You're just bending the lower arm; don't feel that you should hunch your shoulders. They should stay in the comfortable low position of your normal walk.

The elbow remains bent at 90 degrees. Actually, this is the angle only when the arms are hanging directly down from the shoulders. Race walkers want their arms to go forward and back like a piston, with the forearm as parallel to the ground as possible. To keep the forearm parallel to the ground, the angle can close a little when the elbow is back and open a little when your arm is forward.

Step Two

Make your normal walking strides quicker by shortening the length. When your foot isn't on the ground, it's not pushing you forward. In Race Walking, we try to get more push by using a quick stride rhythm.

We can work on lengthening your race walk stride later, but only if we can lengthen it without slowing down the rhythm of your strides. At this stage, if we have to choose between long strides and quick strides, we always choose quick strides with a faster leg turnover rate. The best way to get the feeling of quick strides is to shorten your present strides.

Step Three

Straighten the knee of the leg when it touches the ground.

In races, having a straight leg is one of the two rules, which athletes must observe. Even if you never want to race in your life, the straight leg adds efficiency and power to your action.

There are several cues: choose the one that makes most sense to you until it comes naturally. You can pull your toe back to dorsiflex the foot, in biomechanical terms. Or you can aim to hit the ground with the heel of your leading foot; don't exaggerate the reach forward because this results in overstriding. Or you can tighten your thigh muscles (the quadriceps) as your foot lands.

A useful tip is to concentrate on one side at a time when you first try this action. Most of us have a dominant side, which will just feel easier. It also enables you to focus on the feeling. When you're practicing later, work both sides. For now, just concentrate on the dominant one.

Step Four

Give your arms a good swing. You'll notice how you'll go faster automatically for a few strides. With practice, you'll be able to keep it up for longer. If you're doing it right, you may notice some muscle soreness in the top of your back the next day.

Remember Step One. Keep the elbow bent and swing from the shoulder. Drive your elbow back behind you a little; the other arm will drive forward automatically.

We want short quick strides and short quick arms to match. Imagine a line vertically down the side of your shirt. Don't let the hand go behind that line, nor the elbow go in front of it. Remember, your arms should move parallel to the ground like a piston!

Check whether you are driving forward and back with the shoulder or just flapping your hand and forearm up and down. Of course, you want to drive, not flap.

You may find a tendency for the shoulders to creep up into a shrug. If so, you are not alone. A lot of race walkers do it, especially if they're getting tired. Concentrate on keeping the shoulders low, so that your hand moves at the level of your waist.

Step Five (the Tricky One)

Use your hips more. Ideally, you want to feel that you are driving forward with the hip on each stride. When you are starting out, just focus on the one dominate hip.

The hip forward action is the way race walkers lengthen their stride. By driving the hip forward, you actually carry the leg forward too. When you land, the leg is already directly below your body weight, so less time is spent getting into the right position to drive you forward on each stride.

Doing so is much more effective than simply reaching out with your foot, the normal way in which you might think of lengthening the stride. Reaching out certainly lengthens your stride, but it slows it down too. Sticking your foot out makes you land ahead of your center of mass. You then have to haul all your body weight forward until it is directly above your leg. Only at this point will you start to move ahead again. The delay wastes time and effort on each stride.

This step is tricky because hip mobility varies greatly from person to person. Many of us don't have the mobility in our hips to do that move as easily.

Don't worry if you don't seem to be doing it as well as other people. You can still race walk. A distinct hip motion is the mark of the classic race walk technique. There are plenty of people walking, and competing very well, with less hip action than the classic model. In any event, you don't want an exaggerated hip action to slow you down, however classic it may look.

Once again, the stages of transition from walking to race walking are

1. elbow at 90°
2. shorter, quicker strides
3. straighten leg
4. drive the arm from the shoulder
5. use the hips

If you have race walking friends, you'll probably learn a series of drills we call skill exercises to concentrate on aspects of race walk technique. They can help you with the transition. The exercises are like a musician's scales. You will find them useful for practice or to remind yourself about a specific point of technique.

If you haven't learned the skill exercises, just practice the cues we've described. Rehearse each cue individually and possibly each side individually if you notice a significant difference.

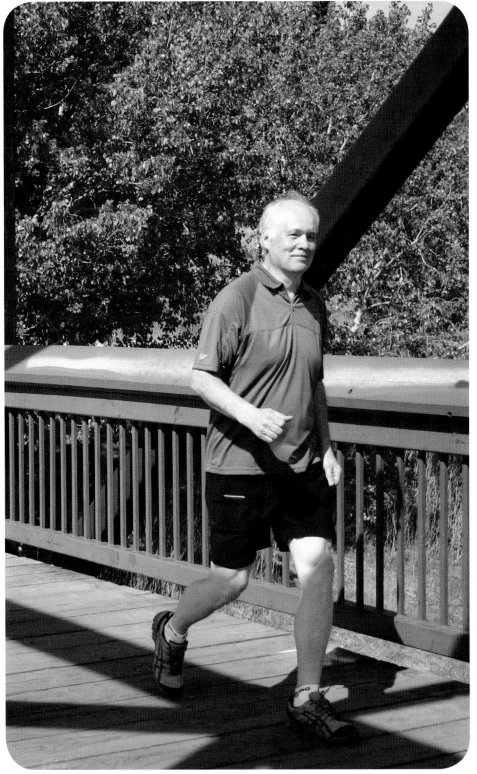

If you practice each stage of the transition over 50 meters, four or five times each with about 30 seconds rest between each repetition, you will find it a good workout in itself. It's a workout that is well worth doing periodically to remind your brain of the proper action you need.

Walking Back to Running

Some participants come to walking programs because they feel that they can't run. They recognize the benefits of walking and are prepared to give it a try because they are inherently active people. Yet there is a tinge of regret that they can no longer run as they used to.

If you are healthy with no medical conditions, the fitness walking program may be able to help. You have simply lost conditioning and strength. When you try to run again, even for a few steps, you feel exertion in your breathing, pain in your joints or both. There may also be a sense of frustration: after all, for example, you were an athlete on your high school cross-country team.

You are suffering the effects of the fourth principle of conditioning, the principle of reversibility. The principle states that a physiological system will revert to previous levels if training loads are not regularly applied. Simply put, use it or lose it.

If your doctor has cleared you to participate in the walking program and unless you are or were a smoker, your major obstacle will be to regain strength in the running muscles of your legs and hips. Working on the postural muscles of your abdomen and back will also make life easier for you. We are going to deal with your return to running by working on strength, at least initially.

This muscular work will be your first priority if you would like to walk or run again. Your cardiovascular system will come along for the ride for the time being.

You need to be on your feet as much as you can. When the program schedule calls for hill walking, consider it tailor-made for you! Definitely walk a few flights of stairs in the office each day, and keep adding a flight or two per day. If you are interested in formal strength work, squats, leg presses and leg curls, our section on resistance training is just what you need. We suggest you keep the weights light and the number of repetitions in your sets at the high end of the range.

Be prepared for some slight soreness in your muscles as they start to carry you again. Keep the soreness to a fulfilling level; it should never restrict your ability to move normally.

When you feel that your strength has improved, you may want to run again. Hold that urge for a while! Get some more strength. You have an intermediate stage to go through. The jump between your present level and the strength you need to run comfortably is too great for you at the moment. Remember that the moment you leave the ground and land again, you are multiplying the impact considerably. As we've discussed elsewhere, the impact is the runner's biggest muscular effort.

Your first walking steps should deliberately be a jog (so that the impact is increased as gradually as possible) and for a few meters only. You need to truly believe that you are doing a resistance exercise—because you are! Each time you land is a repetition, so don't do too many more than you would do in a weight room set. Twenty or so impacts on each leg will take you 40 or 50 meters down the track. That's plenty for now. Rest and do another set. For your first time back running, three sets are fine.

Once you are comfortable with three repetitions, you can increase the number to four or five. When you feel that you could do a few more repetitions with little problem, then you can gradually increase the length of each walk. The pattern of "effort followed by recovery" still applies.

Hill Training

Walking on hills (up and down) has many of the same effects as running on hills. The increased intensity adds to the aerobic benefit. You can reach an anaerobic level on hills too, but let's not yet!

The effort needed to combat gravity is a great way to gain strength, with exactly the same action as we need for our walking. With increased strength comes better, more efficient technique.

Race walkers may also choose to train down the hill. We can increase our stride rate (turnover) to a level difficult to achieve on the flat, which contributes to our skills and our all-important race rhythm. Race walkers should know that they are unlikely to encounter significant hills on a racecourse as they might in a running race. The most you will get is a gentle slope. Maintaining correct technique is no problem walking uphill, but it's virtually impossible going down. Descents are therefore regarded as an unfair obstacle. Since race walk races are held on loops rarely exceeding 2500 meters in length, what goes up must soon come down.

Proper Hill Technique—Going Down

A good number of walkers make walking downhill difficult and risk injury by leaning back and putting on the brakes as they walk down the hill. Here is a tip to improve your walking times and reduce the risk of injury. Gravity is your training buddy. With a slight lean down the hill, gravity will pick up your pace with no additional effort. Many walkers lean back into the hill, but this takes more effort and is slower. Open your stride slightly and lean forward. Come race day the experience of the hill sessions pays big dividends as you pass walkers not only on the uphill but at the crest and on the downhill as well.

Intensity

For those using heart rate to monitor intensity, the target is 80–85% of maximum heart rate. If you are not using heart rate as your gauge of intensity, then pace yourself so that you are walking up the hill as fast as you can without having to stop and rest. Always rest for at least as long as it takes to walk up the hill or until your heart rate is below 120 bpm. Rest is part of your training.

Be careful if you are doing the hill session with a group. Remember, it is not a race but a quality individual workout. Walk to the hill and do the warm-up with the group, but the hill is yours alone to conquer and at your own speed. Hills are magic stuff if treated with respect and some common sense.

Another ingredient that hills add is character. As you do the hill repeats, mentally, or if it helps verbally, repeat the words "character, character." On race day when you discover a hill on the course think back to the hill sessions and the word "character." No race course will have 12 repeats in it. Hills build your confidence level and increase your self-esteem as well as prepare you mentally to be a better athlete.

Training for Women

The body's response to exercise is the same for both sexes. Concerns raised in the past about general inherent risks of women participating in sport have been discredited.

With a few gender-specific exceptions, which we discuss later, women are at no greater risk of injury than men. Injuries occur as a result of stresses to the body, regardless of gender. The key to avoiding them is to adapt the training program to the level of fitness.

Many misconceptions about women's activity come simply from the fact that women have traditionally been compared to men. The fact that women are, in general, smaller than men is a physiological reality. As a criterion of comparative evaluation, it is meaningless! After puberty, women do indeed have generally smaller hearts and lungs and less muscle mass than men. But likewise, each heart and lung and muscle is perfectly adequate for its owner's needs!

Regular exercise offers the same benefits for men and women: greater cardiovascular fitness, muscle tone and bone strength. Fit individuals suffer less sickness and have a positive image of themselves.

Health Concerns for Female Athletes.
Menstruation and Hormonal Changes

Virtually every source of exercise information feels the need to discuss menstruation. These sources, mostly written by men, do not acknowledge that the vast majority of modern women experience their period as a perfectly normal part of their life.

Women experiencing problems, discomfort or any factors that disrupt their normal activity should know that their doctor can likely help. There is no need to suffer in silence.

The problems are rarely related to exercise. Indeed, women often find that exercise, and the associated wellness, actually eases some symptoms of menstrual discomfort.

Elevated levels of exercise can affect the menstrual cycle, especially in women with low body fat. At this point, the exercise is changing the woman's hormone levels in a way that is not desirable and that may have additional consequences.

The reasons are not yet well understood, but it is known that small adjustments to body weight or exercise levels can reverse the problem.

If for any reason periods are irregular, lighter than normal or if they cease entirely, medical advice should be sought. Women who exercise in this situation may well be suffering imbalances and deficiencies, which are a risk factor in conditions such as osteoporosis.

Pregnancy

Most modern obstetricians are delighted if their pregnant clients are active. The stronger muscles and the high levels of fitness generally make for a smoother pregnancy, prepare the woman for the effort of labor and facilitate a return to normal activity levels after delivery.

Every mother-to-be should certainly discuss her exercise routines with her obstetrician, because certain conditions of pregnancy that are classified as high-risk need special attention and care. The doctor needs to know about the athlete's activity and aspirations. The athlete needs to know the medical realities of her case and that of her unborn child.

For most women, the guide to exercise in a normal pregnancy is if you were exercising before you got pregnant, you can continue afterwards until your body tells you differently! Pregnant athletes have continued training, even competed at a high level, with no ill-effect whatsoever. The different stages of pregnancy bring their own limiting factors that will naturally slow you down!

After delivery, the return to activity will take some time, but it is a normal expectation. There will be a period of gentle "training to train" and then a gradual return to previous levels. Some athletes have returned to competition as quickly as four or five months after having a child. Others prefer to take longer.

Significant performance improvement after giving birth is well documented. The exact reasons are not definitively clear. Suggestions range from the physiological (different hormonal levels) to psychological (high fulfillment and a clear sense of life's priorities).

Iron Levels

Together with calcium, iron is one of the few minerals that a normal active person may lack. (Other deficiencies are not normal and need to be assessed medically before indiscriminate supplementation is considered.) Once

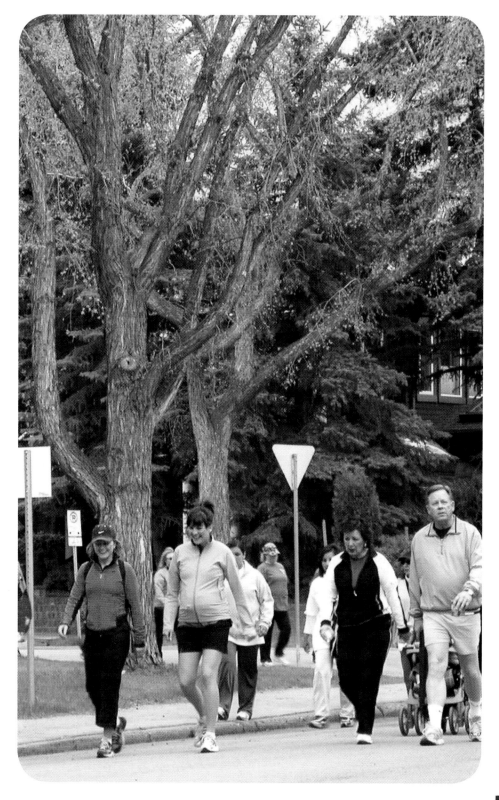

considered exclusively a women's condition, iron deficiency is becoming recognized as a concern for all participants in aerobic activity.

However, women continue to be affected to a higher degree. Studies have shown very high percentages of active women to be iron deficient, often to a debilitating extent. Young active women seem to be less able to absorb dietary iron, and increases with levels of exercise.

Iron is a component of hemoglobin, which circulates in the blood, carrying oxygen to working muscles and tissues. Dietary iron comes in two forms, one more easily absorbed by the body than the other. But neither form is readily absorbed, so conscious attention to iron intake is important, especially for athletes. Restrictive diets of any kind are likely to affect iron levels.

The more accessible heme iron is found in red meat and dark poultry meat. This places vegetarians at even greater risk of deficiency. Non-heme iron, found in fruit, vegetables and grains, is not so easily absorbed.

With low iron levels, less oxygen gets to the working muscles. The result is fatigue, the inability to exercise at previous levels and diminished competitive performance. A doctor seeing a patient with these symptoms will usually suspect low iron levels right away and order the appropriate blood tests. If iron levels drop further, the result is a debilitating condition called anemia.

If you need treatment, the solution is usually iron supplements taken in the form of tablets. A word of caution is necessary. Although iron supplements are available over-the-counter, have your blood tested before taking them. The test will tell your doctor whether you are in the small percentage of the population who will react adversely to the intake of iron supplements.

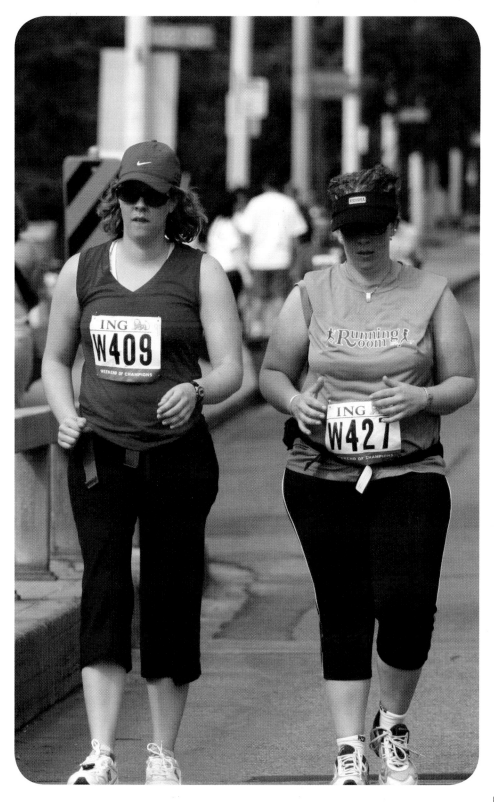

Walking and the Weather

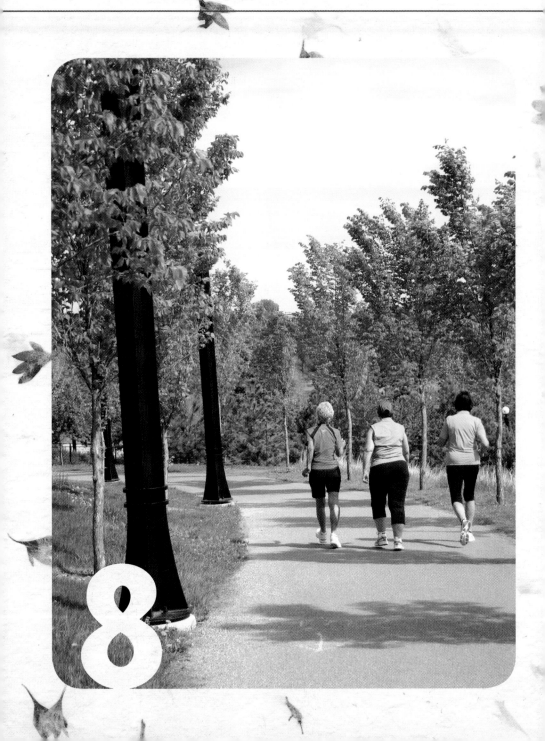

8

Hot Weather Walking

In our North American climate we are often exposed to dramatic temperature changes from hot to cold. This presents us with the challenge of being properly prepared for hot weather walking.

You'll know from your winter holiday to a hot climate that a certain amount of acclimatization to hot weather occurs in just a few days. The heat that blankets you as you leave the plane does not seem so bad by the time you leave your destination. Acclimatization is not immunity; it simply means that your body is automatically taking precautions.

Heat is the one of the endurance athlete's greatest enemies. Heat stress does not need to progress very far before it becomes a medical emergency. It may be unpleasant to contemplate, but heat works on the protein in the body in much the same way as it does on any other protein—it starts to cook!

Luckily, we have defense mechanisms that protect us. Distance athletes may not like the slowing down that these mechanisms produce, but they are there for our protection. At the first sign of any symptoms, stop, cool off and seek medical help.

Your cooling mechanism operates on water. In hot conditions, you need to drink frequently before, during and after exercise. If you feel thirsty, you are already dehydrated. For the length of normal fitness activities, plain water is your most effective drink. Sports drinks work best immediately after you have finished.

Symptoms

Symptoms come in degrees of severity. Heat stress is followed by heat exhaustion, which is followed by heatstroke, a life-threatening condition. These levels are reached as your cooling mechanisms go beyond their capacity.

Heat Stress

Under heat stress, your cooling system is working at the upper limit of its capacity. You will not be able to exercise as vigorously as you can under cooler conditions (but, if you're in a race, neither will any of your competitors). You will be sweating profusely, and you will likely not be enjoying the effort as much as you otherwise might. You will likely feel muscle cramps.

Heat Exhaustion

Heat exhaustion means that your cooling system is overloaded. It is still working, but it is not able to keep up with the cooling demands. Danger is mounting. The body defends you by slowing you down even more, actually trying to make you stop, so that the production of body heat does not continue. The pulse grows weak, you look pale and you may actually feel chills. You begin to feel dizzy and disoriented; your speech slurs, and muscle control is lost.

With rest, fluids and external cooling, the heat-exhausted athlete will recover quite quickly. But the body keeps up its protection as you recover. It doesn't want you to exert yourself for a while. You become very tired and will doze off; your rest is often interrupted by bouts of vomiting. Finally, you will be able to sleep off your experience, likely waking with a wicked headache as a reminder of the stress you were under.

Heatstroke

Heatstroke is when your cooling system simply gives up. If you get heatstroke, you won't remember much about it. You will wake in a hospital bed some time afterwards with an IV in your arm that puts fluids directly back into your body. After a short rest, you will be able to go home. You may wonder what all the fuss was about.

In the meantime, people worked furiously to keep you alive. You stopped sweating. You collapsed and remained unconscious. You were rushed to the hospital and packed in ice, because your body no longer had a way to cool itself. Your body temperature was so elevated that your brain was in danger of being permanently damaged. You were lucky to wake up at all.

Warm-Weather Clothing

This is the time when all you want to do is take it off, but putting something on may keep you cooler and protect you from the sun's harmful rays.

What to wear when the temperature rises:

+ Despite what you have been told, cotton is not the best. Cotton holds moisture, and a lot of it.

+ Exercising in a sweat-soaked cotton shirt on a hot day reduces the ability of water to evaporate from your body. This reduces cooling, particularly in a humid environment.

- Cotton loses its soft texture when wet, which combined with the salt in your sweat, can often cause chafing in places where it comes into contact with the skin.

What to Look for

Look for garments made of synthetics, such as polyester or nylon. These fabrics help to transport moisture from your body to the surface of the fabric, so it can evaporate faster and keep you cool and dry. The more evaporation, the greater the cooling effect on the body.

Remember

- Light-colored garments absorb less light and therefore keep you cooler.
- During bright day conditions, covering up reduces heat accumulation brought on by direct sunlight.
- Wearing fabrics such as CoolMax® Extreme keeps you cooler and dryer and may help reduce summer chafing.
- Wear a hat with a brim. Protect your head from the heat and direct sunlight, especially if you are a man who is a little thin on top.
- Fabric also helps to reduce the exposure of skin to the sun and protects the skin from UV rays. Every fabric has a different rating, but some coverage is better than none!

Is It Safe Out There?

Many factors influence your decision to exercise in hot weather. Acclimatization and hydration aside, there are days, or at least hours during those days, when you shouldn't even try to exercise. When deciding if conditions are safe for strenuous exercise you should refer to the heat index shown on page 145, which combines two conditions, humidity and temperature, to give you the "apparent temperature," or what the heat feels like to your body. If the temperature is 29°C (84°F) and the humidity is 60%, then the apparent temperature is 32°C (90°F). It's something like the wind-chill factor in reverse. But be warned that sunlight is still an important issue. If the air temperature is 29°C (84°F) that means it's 29°C whether it's overcast or sunny. If the sun is out, your body will soak up electromagnetic radiation and heat up much faster than on an overcast day. Treat the figures in the chart as guidelines. It's possible to get heat exhaustion on a 21°C (70°F) day, particularly if you're used to working out in 10°C (50°F) weather.

No matter what climate you're used to or what you're wearing, when the apparent temperature goes over 41°C (105°F), it is best to stay at home—or flee to the nearest air-conditioned fitness center.

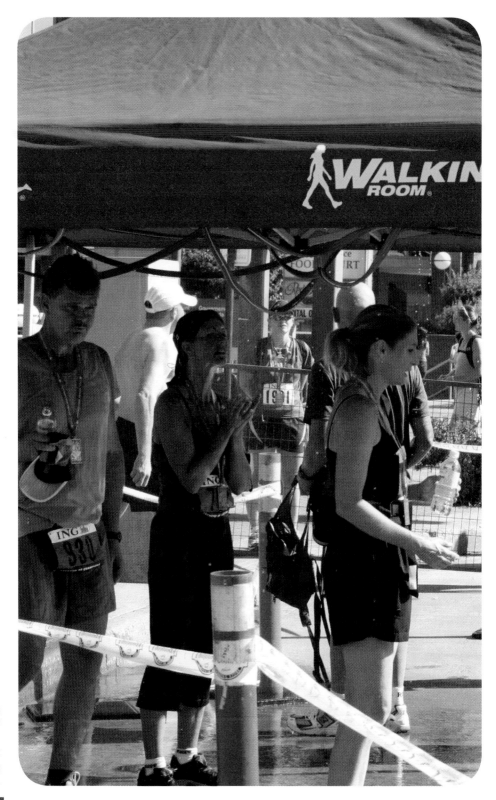

Heat Index

Actual Air Temperature (°C)

Relative Humidity	20	23	26	29	32	35	38	41	44	47	50
Apparent Temperature											
0%	17	20	22	25	28	31	33	35	38	40	43
10%	17	20	23	26	29	32	35	38	41	45	48
20%	18	21	24	27	30	34	37	41	45	50	55
30%	18	22	25	28	32	36	40	45	51	58	65
40%	19	22	25	30	34	38	44	51	59	67	
50%	19	23	27	31	35	42	49	58	67		
60%	20	24	27	32	38	46	56	66			
70%	20	24	29	33	41	51	63				
80%	21	25	29	36	45	58					
90%	21	25	30	38	50						
100%	21	26	32	42							

Actual Air Temperature (°F)

Relative Humidity	70	75	80	85	90	95	100	105	110	115	120
Apparent Temperature											
0%	64	69	73	78	83	87	91	95	99	103	107
10%	65	70	75	80	85	90	95	100	105	111	116
20%	66	72	77	82	87	93	99	105	112	120	130
30%	67	73	78	84	90	96	104	113	123	135	148
40%	68	74	79	86	93	101	110	123	137	151	
50%	69	75	81	88	96	107	120	135	150		
60%	70	76	82	90	100	114	132	149			
70%	70	77	85	93	106	124	144				
80%	71	78	86	97	113	136					
90%	71	79	88	102	122						
100%	72	80	91	108							

Apparent Temperature	Risk from prolonged exercise and/or exposure
18° to 32°C (64° to 90°F)	Fatigue, dehydration possible
32° to 41°C (90° to 105°F)	Heat cramp or heat exhaustion possible
41° to 54°C (105° to 130°F)	Heat cramps or heat exhaustion likely; heatstroke possible
Above 54°C (above 130°F)	Heatstroke very possible

Walking and the Weather

8

Cold Weather Walking

There is a special joy in being the first person to make fresh footsteps in the snow, so don't pass up the excitement of a crisp sunny walk in the early morning or the delight of an evening walk through the darkness as large snowflakes float through the stillness of the evening. Building a snowman in the fresh snow can add a new cross-training regime to your winter workout, so loosen up and enjoy the winter. It's a fact those cold winter days build character—the kind you can use in the late stages of any long walk. If you are feeling rough at any time, think back to the challenges you overcame during those long winter walks.

The following are some cold weather walking tips. Most of the tips involve a common-sense approach to severe conditions.

Cold Weather Tips

1. Adjust the intensity of your workout.

2. A large portion of body heat is lost through the head, so keep it covered.

3. Warm up properly and start your walks at a comfortable pace and slowly build up the pace to a pace slower than your normal training pace.

4. Shorten your stride to improve your footing on icy roads. Wear a pair of slip-on Ice Get A Grips that slip on over the soles of your shoes for greater traction (just like the studded tires on your car).

5. Carry a cell phone.

6. Wind chill does not measure temperature. It measures the rate of cooling. On a day with wind, prepare for the wind-chill factor.

7. Walk into the wind for the first part of your walk and with the wind on the return portion.

8. When walking by yourself walk in a loop around your starting point in case you need to cut the walk short.

9. On your first few walks on snow or ice, you may experience slight muscle soreness in the legs. That is because your supporting muscles are working harder to control your slipping.

10. Cover all exposed skin with clothing or face cream. If you or your walking partner has exposed skin, be aware of each other and the possibility of frostbite.

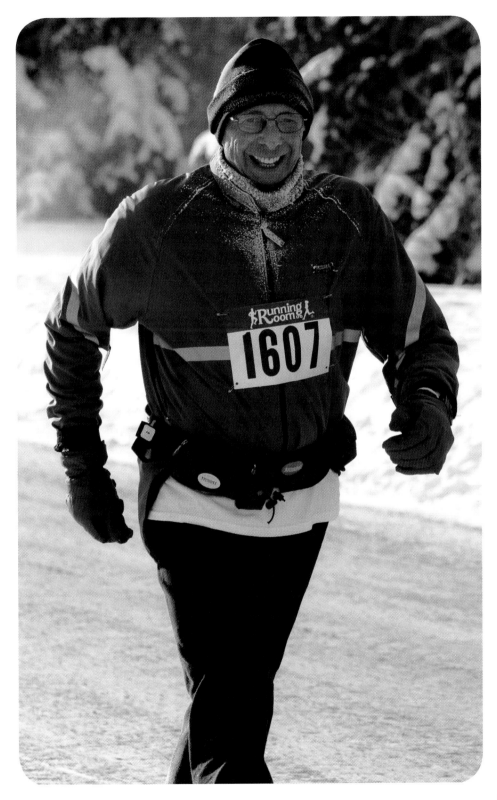

11. In the winter it's dark, so wear reflective clothing or accessories and walk facing the traffic to be more visible.

12. Mittens are warmer than gloves.

13. Drink water on any walk—a sip every 10 minutes.

14. Use a lip balm protector or Body Glide Anti Blister & Anti Chaf on your lips, nose and ears.

15. Gentlemen, wear a wind brief or boxer. Ladies, wear a loose layer over your behind or a winter boxer design to keep you warm.

16. Moisturize your hands to help keep them warm and soft.

17. Walk any speed sessions indoors on a dry surface.

18. Beware of hypothermia for both yourself and those walking with you. This is a drop in your core body temperature. Signs of hypothermia include incoherent slurred speech, clumsy fingers and poor coordination. At the first sign, get to a warm dry place and seek medical attention. You are more likely to experience difficulty on a wet and windy day.

19. Do not accelerate or decelerate quickly in the cold weather.

20. Make sure any changes in direction are gradual to avoid slipping or pulling muscles that are not properly warmed up.

21. Freezing your lungs is just not possible. The air is sufficiently warmed by the body prior to entering the lungs. If you find the cold air uncomfortable, wear a facemask or balaclava to help warm the air.

Winter Clothing

Tips for Dressing in Winter

The key to comfortable cold-weather running is to dress in layers. Air between the layers provides the warmth you feel. Normally, the top half of your body needs three layers and the bottom half two layers to provide warmth.

1. Base Layer
2. Thermal Layer (especially on top half of body)
3. Outer Shell

Base Layer

This is by far the most important layer. If it is doing its job properly, this layer should keep you both warm and dry. Look for form-fitting long-sleeve shirts and long underwear made of technical fabrics that wick moisture and allows evaporation. Cotton is definitely out for this layer because it holds moisture. Keep warm in the winter by staying dry.

Products to look for: Running Room Fit-Wear® base layers made from Thermastat® and Polartec® X-Static.

Thermal Layer

This layer is optional. Not everyone will feel they need the added warmth of this layer. In recent years the development of brushed fabrics like Polar Fleece has made this an additional layer for warmth and not weight, which may be a problem when wearing thick cottons and wools. Do not defeat the purpose of your base layer by using non-technical material. Polartec®Windpro® is a great example of the triple layer fabrics that can act as your base and thermal layers in one.

Products to look for: Running Room Fit-Wear® made from Dryline, Polartec® and WindPro®.

Outer Shell

An outer shell is not a necessity every day but definitely an asset on the colder, windier days. A proper shell should prevent the cold winter wind from reaching your damp base layer as well as allowing moisture and some heat to escape from inside. A windproof, breathable shell is your best bet. Water resistance is an added feature that will allow you to use your investment throughout the entire year.

Products to look for: Running Room Fit-Wear® made from Supermicroft®, Soft Shell, Polartec® and WindPro®.

The following products will help keep you warm, dry and safe:

1. Polartec® X-Static®/ThermaStat base layers
2. Running Room Fit-Wear® top
3. Running Room Fit-Wear® bottom
4. Soft Shell/WindPro® jacket/pants
5. Balaclava
6. Double Layer ThermaStat socks
7. Reflective accessories like battery-powered lights or armbands
8. Reflective vest
9. Energy Bar
10. Angled water bottle carrier

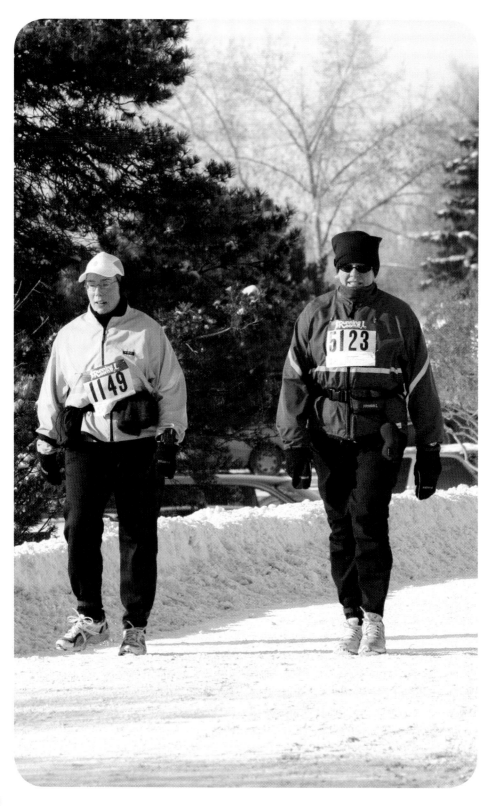

Wind Chill

Actual Air Temperature (°C)

Calm Wind	4	-1	-7	-12	-18	-23	-29	-34	-40
Wind Speed (km/h)	Equivalent Chill Temperature								
8	2	-4	-9	-15	-21	-26	-32	-37	-43
16	-1	-9	-15	-23	-29	-37	-43	-51	-57
24	-4	-12	-21	-29	-34	-43	-51	-57	-65
32	-7	-15	-23	-32	-37	-46	-54	-62	-71
40	-9	-18	-26	-34	-43	-51	-59	-68	-76
48	-12	-18	-29	-34	-46	-54	-62	-71	-79
56	-12	-21	-29	-37	-46	-54	-62	-73	-82
64	-12	-21	-29	-37	-48	-57	-65	-73	-82

Actual Air Temperature (°F)

Calm Wind	40	30	20	10	0	-10	-20	-30	-40
Wind Speed (km/h)	Equivalent Chill Temperature								
5	35	25	15	5	-5	-15	-25	-35	-45
10	30	15	5	-10	-20	-35	-45	-60	-70
15	25	10	-5	-20	-30	-45	-60	-70	-85
20	20	5	-10	-25	-35	-50	-65	-80	-95
25	15	0	-15	-30	-45	-60	-75	-90	-105
30	10	0	-20	-30	-50	-65	-80	-95	-110
35	10	-5	-20	-35	-50	-65	-80	-100	-115
40	10	-5	-20	-35	-55	-70	-85	-100	-115

Apparent Temperature	Risk from prolonged exercise and/or exposure
Above -30° C (-20° F)	Little danger
-30 to -57° C (-20 to -70° F)	Increasing danger—exposed flesh may freeze within 1 minute
Below -57° C (-70° F)	Great danger—exposed flesh may freeze within 30 seconds

Note: Winds above 64 km/h (40 m.p.h.) have little additional effect

8 Walking and the Weather

Heart Rate Monitor Training

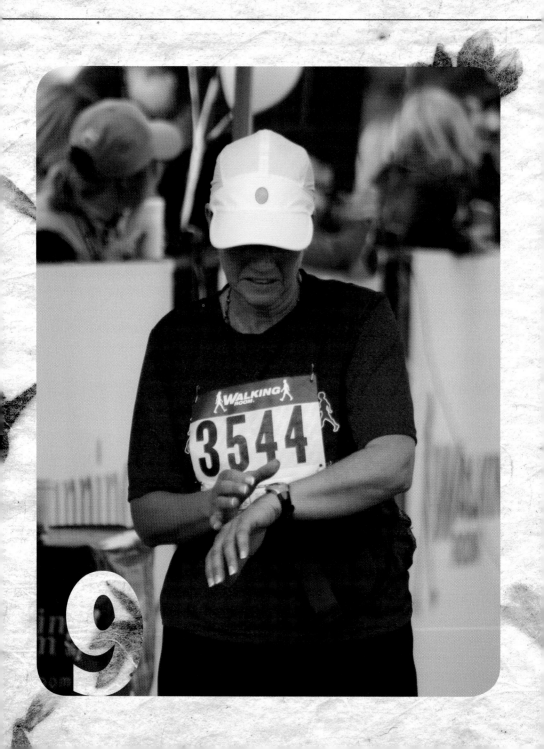

Understanding Exercise Intensity and Target Zones

Different training workouts require you to exercise at different intensities. As your training intensity increases, so does your heart rate. Monitoring your heart rate is probably the most widely known method of determining your training intensity. The development of wireless heart rate monitors has given many athletes, from beginners to experts, an easy and effective way to gauge their training intensity.

You can't always predict how your heart is going to respond to exercise. Fatigue, illness and overtraining can have profound effects on heart rate, so always listen to your body. Don't be a slave to your heart rate monitor; you should look at it about every 10 minutes, not every minute, especially during your training.

Objectives

After completing this chapter you will:

+ understand what exercise intensity is and why it should be measured or tracked during activity
+ determine your estimated maximum heart rate and your personal target heart rate zone for exercise
+ be able to measure how your body responds to cardiovascular activity

The New Tools of the Trade

With a heart rate monitor (HRM), you have at your disposal a powerful control tool for making your workouts more effective and time efficient, safer and—equally important—much more fun.

The Heart Rate Window

Your HRM gives you a physiological window—through accurate heart rate measurement—into your body's response to the moment to moment rigors of physical activity. This precise view of what's happening inside your body allows you to make immediate adjustments in your exercise intensity to the level most appropriate for your body and your particular needs. Far more accurate than any other measure of physical activity—how fast you're going, or how far you've gone, for example—your heart rate reflects exactly how your system is functioning, and provides a measure of how hard you're working. (It's like watching a car's tachometer: The tach tells you how hard your engine's working in revolutions per minute, while your HRM tells you how hard your heart is working in beats per minute.)

9 Heart Rate Monitor Training

More Is Not Better

There is a considerable body of research that tells us that more is not necessarily better when it comes to exercise. In fact, training to exhaustion does far more to hurt performance than to enhance it. A typical adult can still get fit training at far lower levels of intensity than has been traditionally thought. Monitoring your heart rate to keep yourself at the right level of exercise intensity has become the training secret of the decade.

Benefits of Proper Training

Some basic exercises and training goals are universal. For example, strengthening the heart muscle through aerobic activity helps the heart pump more blood with each stroke. As total blood volume increases, the blood becomes better equipped to transport oxygen. Lung capacity increases, blood pressure decreases and the entire cardiovascular system functions more efficiently. Some well-known benefits of aerobic training are better performance, better general health, improved muscle tone, weight loss and relief from stress and insomnia.

Training Smart

Monitoring your heart rate will take the guesswork out of training and ensure that your training intensities are optimal. If your heart rate during exercise is too low, you aren't working hard enough to do yourself much good. If your heart rate is too high, you will most likely fatigue before the exercise can be beneficial. Monitoring your heart rate ensures that you stay within your optimal target heart rate zone, optimizing the benefits of your workouts and eliminating uncertainty about safety.

The Benefits of Monitoring Heart Rate

Heart Rate Monitors and Motivation

Statistics show that over 70% of the people who start an exercise program will quit within the first six months—and many within the first few weeks. What makes it so hard for individuals to stick with an exercise program? Why do they give up so quickly? One of the primary factors affecting adherence to exercise is a loss of motivation.

Most people start an exercise program with a specific goal or need in mind that becomes the driving force or motivation behind their desire to exercise. However, many individuals run into common obstacles that cause them to lose sight of these goals and begin to lose their motivation to keep going.

Fortunately, a heart rate monitor can provide the solution to many of the obstacles that stand in the way of success in an exercise program.

Keeps You in Your Zone

If you want to reach your exercise goals, it's important to stay in your target heart rate zone during workouts. A heart rate monitor is your constant reminder of the intensity and quality of each workout session. Nothing keeps you in your zone more accurately than a heart rate monitor. The Polar© brands of heart rate monitors are some of the best available.

Heart Rate Monitor Shows Your Progress

It takes four to six weeks of consistent exercise before you begin to see any external changes to your body. Although you can't see them, internal improvements begin to take place immediately. Your heart rate is an efficiency rating for your entire body. As your fitness improves, your heart rate improves along with it. A heart rate monitor gives you a physiological window into your body's response to the daily improvements in your physical health.

A Heart Rate Monitor Eliminates Frustration

If your heart rate is too low during exercise, your body reaps little or no benefits. Having a too low heart rate means you're not likely to see the results you want, such as weight loss or increased endurance. If your heart rate is too high during exercise, you may tire too quickly and become frustrated, or even run the risk of injury. In either case, you're likely to quit exercising because you're not getting the results you want or because it's simply too difficult. A heart rate monitor keeps you exercising by showing you results that you otherwise would not see.

Keeps You Safe

Exercising too hard can put you at risk for injury. A heart rate monitor reminds you of the safe and effective heart rate intensity in which you should exercise and warns you when you leave that safety zone.

Exercise Intensity and Heart Rate Monitors

To understand exercise intensity and how a heart rate monitor helps achieve fitness goals, our friends at Polar Heart Rate Monitors provided these rules—be familiar with the three keys to success:

1. Working out at the correct exercise intensity is the only way to achieve your fitness goals.

Too hard = injury, muscle soreness = can't finish workout.

Too easy = no improvement or results = will not reach fitness goals.

2. Heart rate is the only accurate measurement of exercise intensity.

3. Heart rate monitors are the easiest and most accurate way to measure continuous heart rate.

The continuous display of heart rate is what makes your workout effective. This is because your heart rate is guiding you during your whole workout, just like a coach. As the speedometer in your car tells you how fast your car is going, your heart rate tells you how fast and hard you are going.

What Is Exercise Intensity?

Exercise intensity is simply a measurement of how hard you are working at a given time during exercise. The American College of Sports Medicine, the world's leading medical and scientific authority on sports medicine and fitness, recommends that every individual involved in an exercise program should know how hard their body is working during exercise.

Your heart provides key information for determining how intensely you are working during exercise. Your heart rate (how many times your heart beats per minute) is really an efficiency rating for your entire body. The number of times your heart beats during each minute of exercise is a measurement of the intensity of the exercise. If your heart rate is low, exercise intensity is low; if your heart rate is high, your exercise intensity is high.

Why Should Exercisers Monitor Exercise Intensity?

Your heart is the most important muscle in your body and, like all muscles, must be exercised regularly to remain strong and efficient. According to fitness experts, exercise is more effective when you work out in a specific heart rate range or zone. (This is referred to as your Target Heart Rate Zone, TZ.) This zone can vary greatly depending on your age, fitness level and various other factors.

Example

Debby and Thomas are at the same cardiovascular fitness level and plan to compete in a 5 mile event. Debby decides to walk briskly and Thomas decides to sprint. Whose exercise intensity level will allow them to maintain their speed for the entire 5 miles? The answer is Debby. Thomas will be too tired to sprint the entire 5 miles; he cannot maintain exercise intensity that high.

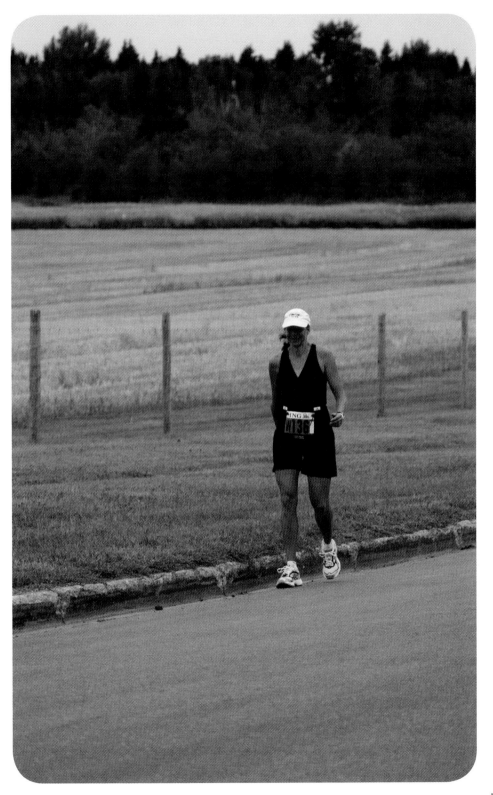

Monitoring exercise intensity helps you stay at a level of exercise that allows you to accomplish your goals. In fact, the ACSM recommends that, in order to get the most benefits from your cardiovascular exercise, you should work within your TZ for at least 20–60 minutes per workout, three to five times per week, at an intensity of 60–80% of your maximum heart rate. Knowing your exercise intensity (heart rate) will allow you to work at the right level of exercise to accomplish this.

What Is Maximum Heart Rate?

Maximum heart rate (MHR) is the maximum attainable heart rate your body can reach before total exhaustion. True maximum heart rate is measured during a fatigue or stress test. This test must be done in a clinical setting and is not practical or accessible for most people. Fortunately, your maximum heart rate can be estimated with a high degree of accuracy using the following simple formula:

Male Estimated Maximum Heart Rate = 220 – Your Age
Female Estimated Maximum Heart Rate = 226 – Your Age
If John is 30 years old, what is his estimated maximum heart rate?
John's Estimated Maximum Heart Rate = 220 – 30
John's Estimated Maximum Heart Rate = 190

John's heart can beat an estimated maximum of 190 times per minute before his body would tire or "max out." This number is extremely helpful because it tells us the absolute highest exercise intensity John can handle before his body wears out. What this means is that during exercise, John should keep his heart rate below his maximum so that he will not become exhausted and have to quit. In fact, this gives John a specific percentage range of his maximum heart rate to exercise in, known as his Target Heart Rate Zone (TZ).

How Do I Determine My Target Heart Rate Zone?

Your Target Heart Rate Zone represents the minimum and maximum number of times your heart should beat in one minute of exercise. The ACSM recommends that all individuals should work within a TZ of 60–80% of their maximum heart rate (MHR). This means that your heart rate during exercise should not fall below 60% or rise above 80% of your maximum heart rate. Let's look at John from our earlier example.

John is 30 years old, so his estimated maximum heart rate is 220 – 30 or 190 beats per minutes (bpm). The ACSM says that John should exercise between

60% and 80% of 190 bpm to stay in his TZ. Let's determine John's TZ:

John will want to keep his heart rate in the range of 114–152 bpm during exercise in order to achieve his goals. If John is a beginning exerciser, he'll want to stay at the low end of his TZ. If John is a more advanced exerciser, he may want to work at the higher end of his TZ to challenge himself more.

In summary, to define your TZ:
- the level that your heart rate needs to get to = lower limit
- the level that your heart rate should not exceed = upper limit
- keeping your heart rate between the lower and upper limits = staying within your TARGET ZONE

The Formula to Find Your Target Zone:
220 minus your age = maximum heart rate (MHR)
MHR x 60% = lower target zone limit
MHR x 80% = upper target zone limit

The Importance of Target Heart Rate Zone (TZ) in the Workout
Staying within your TZ is critical to meeting your exercise goals. However, the question becomes, "What is the correct TZ?" Before that question can be answered, you must know what your exercise goal is, because the most effective TZ is matched with your exercise goal.

- maintain or lose weight, your TZ is 60–70% of MHR
- reach cardiovascular fitness, your TZ is 70–80% of MHR
- increase athletic performance, your TZ is 80% + of MHR

John's Estimated MHR	=	190 bpm
190 bpm (MHR) x 0.60 (60%)	=	114 bpm
190 bpm (MHR) x 0.80 (80%)	=	152 bpm
John's TZ	=	114–152 bpm

Base Training (Recovery/Endurance)
Foundation

Typically, you should find it difficult to keep your heart rate below the limits you have set for yourself. Don't cheat! Strict training in this area will prevent you from losing steam the last few kilometers of your long walk. All training at this level is done at 60–70% of your maximum heart rate.

Threshold (Aerobic) Training
Building the Walls

A good guideline in most cases is to walk at your 5K race pace. The purpose of this type of training is to work on proper form, strength and endurance. Hill training qualifies in this part of the house. Like hill training, you are not going to do this type of walk every day. Any more than a couple times per week will over fatigue your legs and compromise your long walk. All training at this level is done at 70–80% of your maximum heart rate.

Speed Training (Anaerobic)
Putting on the Roof

Remember, owing to their intensity, walks of this nature are best done as interval training. Your intervals should be no longer than a few minutes. Your heart rate should recover to approximately 120 bpm (one to two minutes of rest) before starting the next interval. Like hills, start off with only a few (two to three). Vary the distances of each interval and the total distance covered from week to week. Build slowly from there. With this type of training, a warm-up and cool down are critical. The athlete should warm up with a couple of kilometers of easy walking and a stretch. All training at this level is done at a range of 80% plus of your maximum heart rate.

Skill & Technique Phase
80% Plus Maximum Heart Rate
- 5K to 10K race pace
- Speed intervals
- Increased athletic performance

ANAEROBIC

Strength & Endurance Phase
Hill Training/Tempo/Fartlek
Done at 70–80% Maximum Heart Rate
- These walks should be at a pace where you can talk, but not easily
- Approaching anaerobic threshold but staying just below it
- Reach cardiovascular fitness

Base Training
Steady Runs & Long Slow Distance (LSD) Runs
Done at 60–70% Maximum Heart Rate
- These walks should be easier, and you are still able to carry on a conversation
- Maintain or lose weight

AEROBIC

RECOVERY ENDURANCE

Aerobic or Anaerobic? That is the Question

These terms are thrown around quite loosely in gyms and on the track these days. Here's the low-down on what they really mean. Aerobic means "in the presence of oxygen." What makes an activity aerobic or not is its intensity. Energy for low-intensity exercise can be supplied by aerobic metabolism. Although aerobic metabolism can supply a lot of energy (from birth to death), it can only do so quite slowly. Aerobic metabolism is very efficient and has very few by-products such as lactic acid. Only very small amounts of lactic acid are produced during aerobic exercise. The body can normally remove this before we feel any adverse effects.

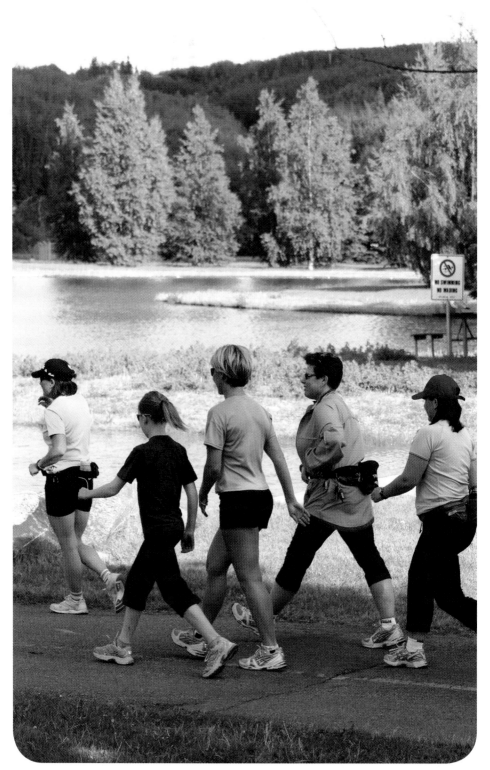

During high-intensity exercise there is a quick and high demand for energy at a very fast rate. Since aerobic metabolism is too slow to supply the energy, our body must shift gears and produce energy at a faster rate. Although anaerobic metabolism can produce a lot of energy in a very short time, the chemical reactions involved create a great amount of lactic acid. So much lactic acid is produced that we cannot get rid of it fast enough, causing it to accumulate in the muscles and blood. Lactic acid accumulation to a high level causes that burning feeling in the legs and queasy feeling in the stomach. If anaerobic exercise persists, lactic acid interferes in the energy-making process. Exercise intensity will have to slow in order to continue or come to a complete halt. This is why predominantly anaerobic exercise can be done for no longer than approximately two minutes. Yes, only two, even for highly trained athletes. For most of us, it's less!

Examples of Predominantly Aerobic Exercise:
+ Walking
+ Running easy
+ Cycling easy
+ Swimming

Anaerobic means "in the absence of oxygen"; when the intensity of exercise is too high for the body to get enough oxygen, and aerobic metabolism is too slow to supply energy at such a fast rate, the body must shift gears and produce energy by anaerobic metabolism. Such high-intensity exercise is called anaerobic exercise.

Examples of Predominantly Anaerobic Exercise:
+ Speed work, as outlined in *Chapter 4, Developing Your Walking Program.*

No one activity is only aerobic or only anaerobic. Most activities that we participate in day to day require both types of metabolism.

Glossary of Heart Rate Terms

Resting Heart Rate
It is the number of times your heart beats per minute during complete uninterrupted rest. It is usually taken upon waking in the morning, before you lift your head from the pillow.

Maximum Heart Rate
It is the highest number of times your heart can contract in one minute. It can

only be measured accurately by taking a stress test in which you exercise until exhaustion. Predictive formulas are most commonly used.

A more practical test for maximal heart rate without a stress test is the maximal hill walk. To perform this test you need the following:

1. a hill (6–8% grade, approx. 400–600 m in length)
2. heart rate monitor
3. a healthy dose of determination

After an appropriate warm-up of at least 10 minutes, which includes stretching, make your way to the bottom of the hill you have chosen. From there you walk as hard as you can without stopping, to the top. At the top, check your heart rate monitor. You should be pretty close to your maximum heart rate. Don't stop at the top. You have just walked really hard and taxed your anaerobic system, so there will be a lot of lactic acid in your blood and muscles. An active recovery of slow gentle walking will speed your recovery and help remove lactic acid from your muscles and blood. Be sure to do a proper cooldown, including some stretches.

Anaerobic Threshold

This threshold is the point (intensity, heart rate, speed) at which aerobic metabolism is not able to supply energy fast enough to keep up with the demands of the activity. A shift to anaerobic metabolism takes place and, if continued, exercise will cease (whether you want it to or not).

VO2 Max

This is the maximum amount of oxygen our muscles can use for exercise. Our bodies are able to take in much more oxygen than our muscles could ever use. What we do by endurance training is train our heart, lungs and blood to deliver more oxygen to the exercising muscles. We also train our muscles to use more oxygen more efficiently. VO2 max occurs at the intensity of exercise that corresponds to maximum heart rate. We are usually able to exercise at this intensity for only a few minutes.

Anaerobic Threshold Heart Rate (ATHR)

This threshold is the heart rate that corresponds with the change from aerobic to predominantly anaerobic metabolism. The threshold is often known as OBLAS: onset of blood lactate accumulation.

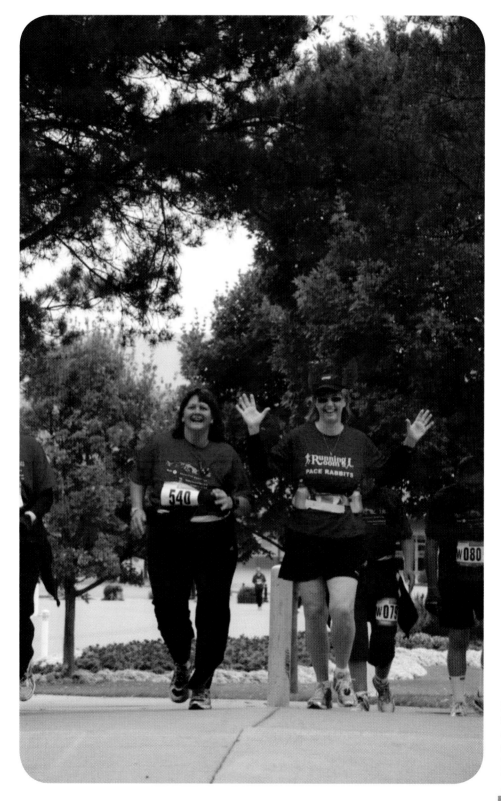

Heart Rate Monitor Training

Heart Rate Recovery

This is the time after you exercise that is used to measure the reduction in your heart rate. Total heart rate recovery is the time between cessation of exercise and return to normal heart rate. A common recovery time is two minutes.

Calculate Heart Rate Training Zones

Using Heart Rate Reserve (HRR) to calculate your heart rate training zones is also referred to as the Karvonen method. The formula is HRR x Intensity% + HR minimum (resting heart rate).

To calculate your HRR take your HR max (maximum heart rate)— 226 minus age for women or 220 minus age for men—and subtract your resting heart rate. You can then use that in the formula above to calculate the following zones:

Zone 1: 50–60%
Zone 2: 61–70%
Zone 3: 71–80%
Zone 4: 81–90%
Zone 5: 91–100%

Remember, the best time to measure your resting heart rate is just as you wake or just before you go to sleep. Your heart rate (both at rest and in training) can be elevated by many factors, including:

+ stress (work, emotional, etc.)
+ nutrition, especially hydration levels
+ heat (until your body adapts to it, usually in 7–12 days)
+ altitude (you will have a higher HR for the same level of intensity at higher elevations, so give your body three weeks or so to adapt)

Recording Heart Rate Information

Resting Heart Rate (RHR)

Heart rate is expressed as beats per minute (bpm). The RHR is a person's heart rate at rest—the lowest number of heartbeats per minute at complete rest.

The best time to find out your resting heart rate is in the morning, after a good night's sleep, and before you get out of bed.

On average the heart beats about 60–80 times a minute when we're at rest, but for top athletes it can be below 30 bpm. RHR usually rises with age, and it generally decreases as your fitness level increases.

RHR is used to determine one's training Target Heart Rate (THR). Athletes sometimes measure their RHR as one way to find out if they're overtrained. An exceptionally high RHR may be a sign of over-exertion or illness.

Average Heart Rate (AHR)

The Average Heart Rate (bpm) figure is a calculation of your average heart rate during your last workout. You can use this measurement to determine the effectiveness of your exercise program and see your progress.

Target Heart Rate (THR)

THR is a range of heart rates that a person chooses to aim for when exercising, based on their personal fitness goals. Target heart rate zones are expressed as percentages of a person's maximum heart rate (MHR). Target heart rate lets you measure your initial fitness level and monitor your progress in a fitness program. For a rough estimate of your maximum heart rate (MHR) subtract your age from 220. For first-time exercisers, have your physician perform a stress test to determine your MHR along with your target zones specific to your goal. This is especially important if you are just starting an exercise program or have not exercised for a prolonged period of time.

Why is establishing daily THR so important?

The most effective way to reach your fitness goal is to exercise in your target heart rate zone. There is a target zone that's right for each day's workout. For example, if you want to improve aerobic fitness you need to be working at 70–80% of your MHR, for 40–60 minutes per day, three to four times per week. Without this information, you would get on a treadmill and not know how hard or how long you should be exercising. In most cases you may be going too easy or too hard. Our friends at Polar Electro (specialist in heart rate monitors) have suggested the following guidelines:

There are three key target zones that will help you achieve specific goals.

60–70%	Lose Weight or Recover
70–80%	Improve Aerobic Fitness
80+ %	Increase Athletic Performance

Sample Training Programs Based on Heart Rate Zones

In this section we have provided four sample workouts that use heart rate as the foundation. We start out with a simple easy steady walk program that keeps your HR consistent at 50–60% MHR. We then move to another program that establishes a MHR threshold at 60–70% MHR, which is the best fat burning level. The next two programs will start to challenge you to improve aerobic fitness and to increase athletic performance by setting MHR levels to achieve peak anaerobic benefit at 80% plus MHR.

Easy Steady Walk

The steady walk can be done daily, or used as a recovery day for alternating with other walking workouts.

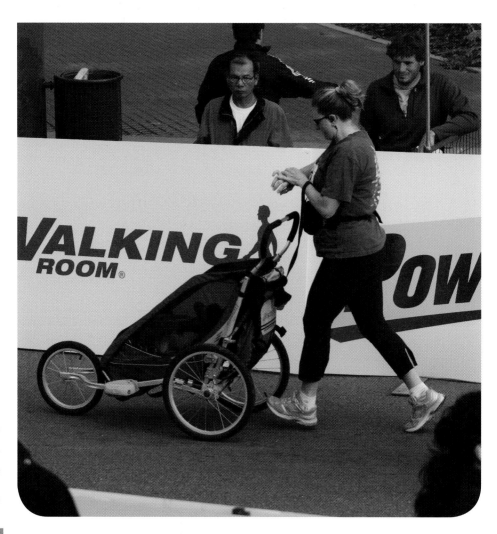

+ Start at an easy pace for 5–10 minutes.
+ Continue walking at a pace that brings your heart rate up to 50–60% of your maximum heart rate (MHR).
+ Walks at a comfortable pace where you can carry on a full conversation comfortably although you may be breathing harder than usual.
+ Walk for 30–60 minutes.
+ End with five minutes of a nice easy stroll or recovery walk. A gentle stretch is recommended as well.

Benefits

This workout builds long-term health and well being. Medical studies have shown an association between walking 30–60 minutes daily and the reduced risk of cancer, heart disease, stroke, type II diabetes and gall bladder disease. It is also associated with increased longevity and decreased risk of hip fracture in those over 60.

Lose Fat and Lose Weight Walk

The fat burning walk can be done daily, or used as a recovery day for alternating with other walking workouts. Those wanting to lose body fat should do this walk most days of the week.

Fat Burning Walking Workout

+ Start at an easy pace for 10 minutes (this burns off the stored blood sugar and glycogen and tells the body to get ready to burn fat).
+ Walk 30–60 minutes at a pace that brings your heart rate up to 60–70% of your maximum heart rate (MHR).
+ This is a comfortable pace where you can speak in full sentences although you will be breathing harder than usual.
+ Cool down with 5–10 minutes at an easy pace.
+ End with five minutes of a nice easy stroll or recovery walk. A gentle stretch is recommended as well.

Benefits

This workout gets the body to use stored fat for energy. At 60–70% of your maximum heart rate, 85% of your calories burned are fats. Walking faster or slower burns a smaller percentage of fat.

Improving Your Aerobic Fitness Walk

You should do this workout every other day. On the days in between, do the steady walk or the fat-burning walk.

Workout

* Start at an easy pace for 5–10 minutes.
* Continue walking at a pace that brings your heart rate up to 70–80% of your maximum heart rate (MHR).
* This is a quick pace where you are breathing hard and able to speak in short sentences.
* Walk for 30–50 minutes at this pace.
* Cool down with 5–10 minutes at an easy pace.
* End with five minutes of a nice easy stroll or recovery walk. A gentle stretch is recommended as well.

Benefits

This walk improves aerobic fitness by increasing the number and size of blood vessels in the muscles and increasing your lung power. At this intensity, 50% of your calories burned are fats, 1% are proteins and 50% are carbohydrates. The aerobic phase of your workout should be of 50 minutes or less to prevent build-up of lactic acid.

Anaerobic Threshold Walk

You should do this workout one to three times per week, alternating with an easier walk day or a rest day.

Workout

* Start at an easy pace for 5–10 minutes.
* Continue walking at a pace that brings your heart rate up to 80–90% of MHR for no more than 50 minutes.
* This is a fast pace where you are breathing very hard and can only speak in short phrases.
* End with five minutes of a nice easy stroll or recovery walk. A gentle stretch is recommended as well.

Benefits

This walk increases your athletic performance by bringing your body up to the anaerobic threshold. It is used by race walkers to improve their VO2 maximum (the highest amount of oxygen one can consume during exercise). It improves endurance.

Warning Signs of Trouble

The symptoms listed below are warnings that more serious trouble might develop if you don't take immediate preventive action. Develop a sensitive eye to these signals. By quickly interpreting and acting upon these symptoms, you can stop trouble at its source:

- resting pulse rate significantly higher than normal when taken first thing in the morning
- sudden, dramatic weight loss
- difficulty falling asleep or staying asleep
- sores in and around the mouth and other skin eruptions
- any symptom of a cold or the flu (sniffles, sore throat or fever)
- swollen, tender glands in the neck, groin or underarms
- dizziness or nausea before, during or after training
- clumsiness—tripping or kicking yourself—during a run over even smooth ground
- any muscle, tendon or joint pain or stiffness that remains after the first few minutes of walking

Nutrition

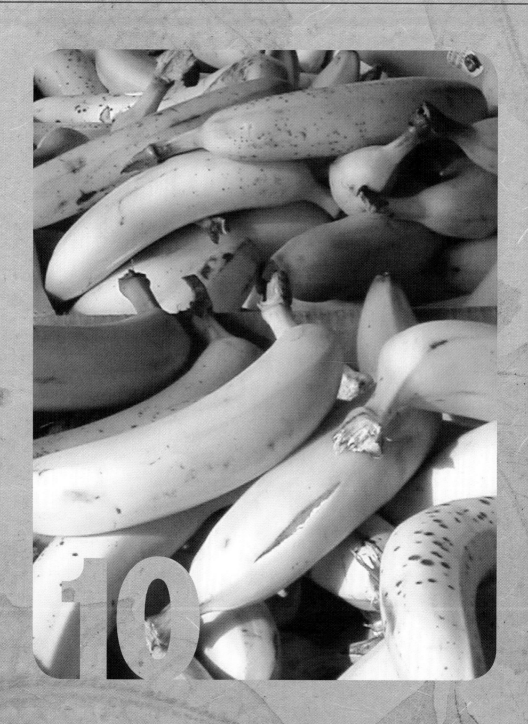

10

Introduction

There are literally hundreds of books dedicated to the topics of nutrition and weight control. The following pages should provide you with appropriate guidelines for healthful eating while participating in an active lifestyle.

Walking for Weight Loss

Macronutrients

Macronutrients are the main components of food that the body needs on a chemical level. There are five macronutrients:

+ carbohydrates
+ fats
+ proteins
+ vitamins and minerals
+ water

Water is such an important nutrient in an endurance athlete's life that it has a section of its own.

There is no magic involved or one diet that everyone can follow for optimal energy and a trim waistline. As individuals we have different energy requirements. Energy requirement is a product of our activity level, body composition, body size and perhaps genetics. There is one thing common to all individuals—food is energy. There are three main sources of energy: carbohydrates, proteins and fats. Healthful eating requires that we take in adequate amounts of all these energy sources.

Carbohydrates

Carbohydrates are the best source of energy, ideally making up 55–65% of your total energy intake. There are two types of carbohydrates—simple and complex. Once digested, both types are used in the form of glucose. Carbohydrates can be stored in the muscle and in the liver in the form of glycogen.

Simple forms such as those found in sugar and fruit are absorbed quickly into the bloodstream. If taken in large quantities, these foods give you a sugar high followed immediately by a sugar low or crash. The sugar high can provide quick energy, but the low is associated with a feeling of lethargy and sometimes even nausea.

Complex carbohydrates are found in foods such as pasta, potatoes, cereals and breads. They are slow-absorbing, providing the body with a slower, steadier stream of glucose.

If the rate of sugar absorption is a medical concern to you, your doctor or nutritionist will show you how to check each food's Glycemic Index, a scientific scale of absorption rate. Choose the foods with a Glycemic Index that your medical situation requires.

Fats

We cannot live without a certain amount of fat. Of all the macronutrients, fat's main function is to be stored. Once stored, it fulfills a variety of other useful functions. Our modern storage needs are reduced because, unlike our remote ancestors, we know where our next meal is coming from. Fat needs only be a comparatively small part (30% or less) of our energy intake. In our North American diet, this is rarely a problem. The primary dietary fats are saturated and unsaturated.

Saturated fats are found in animal products, such as cheese, butter, meat and poultry. In many cases, these fats are visible because they are solid at room temperature.

Unsaturated fats are found in plant sources. There are two types of unsaturated fat. Monounsaturated fat is found in olive, canola and peanut oils and avocados. Polyunsaturated fats are found in sources, such as safflower and sunflower oils, as well as in certain types of fish, such as salmon, tuna and sardines.

Cholesterol is a fat that is often feared because of its links to cardiovascular disease. A small amount of cholesterol is essential to many functions in the body. Cholesterol is produced by the body as well as being obtained in the diet. Sources include animal products, such as eggs, organ meats and shrimp. A diet high in saturated fat may raise cholesterol levels.

Proteins

Proteins are made of 21 different amino acids, which are the building blocks of the human body. When the body is in need of regeneration or repair, such as after training, amino acids provide the raw material. The amino acids that the body can produce are known as nonessential. The others, known as essential amino acids, must be provided by the diet.

Proteins containing all the essential amino acids are known as complete proteins. Animal products, such as meat, eggs and milk products, are great sources of complete proteins. However, they also tend to be higher in saturated fat and cholesterol. These sources should be used in moderation. But by choosing lean cuts of meat and low fat dairy products, they are a valuable part of a healthy diet.

Proteins missing one or more of the essential amino acids are known as incomplete proteins. Sources are cereals, legumes and nuts. Combinations of incomplete proteins can provide all essential amino acids. Vegetarians need to be especially concerned with taking in complete proteins.

In most North American diets, lack of protein is rarely a concern. Excess protein causes water retention and associated urinary complications. High protein foods also tend to be associated with high levels of fat.

Vitamins and Minerals

Vitamins cannot be made in adequate quantities by the body, so they must be provided in the diet. Vitamins play a key role in growth and cellular function. Vitamin levels are normally self-regulating, and there is generally no need to worry unless you experience specific symptoms of a deficiency (too little) or toxicity (too much) of a particular vitamin.

Minerals are also important for cell function and provide materials for structures such as bones and teeth. The major minerals that active people need to ensure in their diet are iron (a component of hemoglobin, the oxygen transporter in the blood) and calcium (important in the maintenance of bone tissue and the prevention of conditions associated with bone tissue loss).

The market is full of nutritional supplements that promise vitamins and minerals to enhance your lifestyle. It is easy to be confused by the amount of information available.

A balanced diet based on Canada's Food Guide should provide a healthy person with all the nutrients you need, including vitamins and minerals. Beyond that, consider supplementation to be a medical matter, not an aid to your training. Deficiencies can sometimes arise for different reasons. Your doctor can identify any concerns specific to you and a nutritionist will help you to solve the problem. General supplementation is not likely to do anything for you that a healthy balanced diet will not do, except lighten your wallet.

Physical Activity and the Vegetarian

It is, of course, possible to be physically active without eating meat. However, the vegetarian should be aware of factors in the diet that must be addressed in order to accommodate the activity. When in doubt, check with a nutritionist who will assess your particular situation.

The more committed to complete vegetarianism you are, the greater your need for attention to your food intake.

As described in the section on proteins, reduced intake of meat means a reduced intake of the amino acids that build the various kinds of proteins in our bodies. Meat, dairy and soy products contain all the essential amino acids. Protein in other vegetables and legumes is called incomplete because some amino acids are present only in low levels. Incomplete proteins can be combined to provide all amino acids, but you need to know the combinations.

A reduced intake of meat, especially red meat, means that your iron intake is almost certainly lower than you need. Iron is a vital component in the production of aerobic energy. Iron in vegetables, even green leafy vegetables, is not easily absorbed. If you are a vegetarian, you will need to know where your iron supply is coming from.

Vegetarians seeking weight loss should also be aware that their diet may not automatically provide it. Active people are hungry people: a vegetarian's intake of calories may actually be high as you chow down on your rice, your granola and your pasta. Some supposed protein replacements have a high-fat content (cheese, beans, nuts). Remember, fat's main job is to be stored!

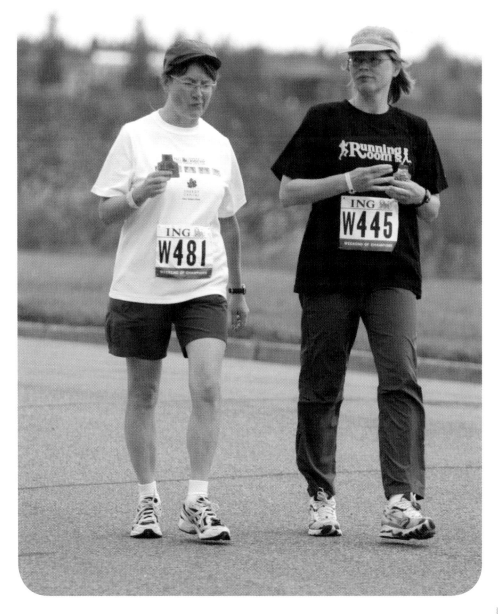

The Scale

Do yourself a favor today and give your scale away, preferably to someone you don't like. Let the scale in your doctor's office manage your health. For the most part, it is only an accurate measure of how much water we have consumed and whether or not we are well hydrated.

Rather than using a scale to chart your progress, take some measurements of your chest, arms, thighs, calves, hips and waist. Mark them down and revisit the measurements every couple of months.

An even simpler way to see our body change is to get a tight pair of pants, one that you can just barely stuff yourself into, and mark them. Those pants will be your benchmark of fitness today and into the future. Once a week, try on the pants to see how they fit.

Alternately, for those of you who are brave and not particularly concerned about modesty, stand naked in front of a mirror. What you see today is the start point. Once a week, make your trip to the full-length mirror. I do suggest that this be done alone; the mirror can be blatantly honest, and this is not the time for family critics.

Weight Control: an Understanding and That's All

The Calorie

A calorie is a measure of heat energy. Strictly speaking, we get the word wrong in daily life. The unit we all know as a calorie is, to scientists, actually a kilocalorie, the amount of heat necessary to raise the temperature of one liter of water by one degree Celsius. We'll use the commonly understood word calorie in this booklet.

An average-sized person needs about 1700 calories per day to maintain basic metabolism (the energy needs of staying in bed all day!). About a fifth of that goes to the brain. The hardworking liver takes almost a third. The heart takes surprisingly little (10%). Any activity adds to the calorie needs at a rate that varies with intensity. A brisk walk uses about five calories per minute. Pick up the pace, or start to stroll, and you double that to 10 calories per minute.

In nutrition, calories measure (a) the energy value of the food we eat and (b) the effort we expend in our daily activity. We should not make the common mistake of seeing the calorie as a measure of nutritional value. A piece of cardboard has a caloric content. But it doesn't fit into any of the essential food groups!

As we discussed previously, we should pay most attention to the macronutrients the food gives us. The nutritional value of our food is, in most cases, a more important concern for us than the amount of calories the food contains.

Any nutrition professionals helping us will very likely pay most attention to the composition of our caloric intake before they worry about the actual number of calories. In most cases, we do not need to be counting calories, unless we are asked to by a health professional for a specific reason. This reason will be either to establish a simple balance between caloric intake and caloric output or to correct a clear imbalance.

Maintenance of body weight: Energy Intake = Energy Output

This equation is one case where an understanding of calories helps with a problem that millions of people wrestle with daily—their body weight.

If you are assessed to be significantly overweight as you begin an exercise program, it is likely that you will lose weight as a result of the exercise. If your bodyweight is in a more normal range, exercise may not actually cause you to lose weight. Many factors of your basic body composition are genetically determined.

Nutrition

But you will be pleased with the changes in your body. You will almost certainly shed some unnecessary fat, but you will also gain muscle tissue, which is firm and attractive by comparison to the fat you are losing (but heavier). You will gain muscle tone and your posture will improve. Above all, remember the real changes that are going on deep beneath the surface as your cardiovascular system improves.

If we get comfortable with the energy intake/output equation, we can spend less time worrying about details of body weight and more time on more important concerns: the nutritional value of the food we eat and the overall benefits of our fitness program.

It really comes down to simple math.

Hydration

Modern sport drinks all contain the fluids necessary for replacement. Many athletes find them appetizing and refreshing. This is a matter of personal taste. The nutrient value is generally less than that of fruit juices and solid replacement food.

The purpose of drinking fluids is to replace water. We are constantly losing water during exercise, we lose it in great quantities. Almost any drink that you find appetizing, even carbonated ones if they are to your taste, will re-hydrate you. The exception is drinks containing alcohol or caffeine, which have a diuretic effect. If you enjoy coffee or a beer, balance it with at least the same amount of other fluid to maintain your hydration.

But do not consider water replacement to be the same as recovery nutrition. Even the most fashionable sport drink should be considered no more than a pleasant tasting appetizer until you feel ready for a decent meal. Recovery snacks such as fruits, bagels, yogurt and cereal do a better job of replacing the nutrients you need as part of your recovery from exercise.

How Much Is Enough?

Endurance walking dramatically increases your need for water and other fluids. You may have heard that you should take in 8 cups (2 L) of fluid each day for good health. However, what many people do not realize is that this recommendation describes the minimum amount of fluid required by an inactive person. It does not account for prolonged activity and is far too low to meet the needs of marathon and half marathon walkers.

Significant amounts of body water can be lost during the course of a long walk. Sweat losses of 500 ml (two cups) of body water per hour are not unusual. These losses must be replaced or physical performance will drop off.

More is better when it comes to taking in enough fluids. Healthy, active people are unlikely to overdo it with fluids. If you are someone who is currently not drinking much you may need to focus on this aspect of nutrition for a while in order to change your behavior. Keep the following guidelines in mind to make sure that you are getting enough fluid:

+ Drink regularly when you are not active—sip 125 ml (½ cup) to 250 ml (1 cup) per waking hour of your day.
+ Center some of your fluid intake around your walks or other activities.
+ Drink 500 ml (two cups) of fluid in the two-hour period before exercise.
+ Take time out to drink 150 ml (⅔ cup) to 300 ml (1⅓ cups) of fluid every 20 minutes during exercise.

What Counts as Fluid?

In general, all decaffeinated, nonalcoholic beverages contribute to your daily fluid intake. This includes water, sparkling water, caffeine-free teas and coffee, fluid replacement sport drinks, juices and milk.

Some liquids can actually promote dehydration. Consume regular coffee and teas, caffeinated soft drinks and alcoholic beverages in moderation to avoid this effect.

Do I Need to Use Sport Drinks?

Sport drinks or fluid/electrolyte replacement beverages help to "top up" blood glucose levels. This, in turn, helps to preserve or spare your glycogen stores and promote endurance. Sport drinks also replace minerals like potassium and sodium that are lost during exercise. Research indicates that during prolonged activity (i.e., more than one hour of activity) these products may improve performance. Not all walkers can tolerate sport drinks. Recognizing this, it is important to experiment with sport drinks during training to assess their impact on your individual performance. Never try a sport drink on race day if you have not already tested it during training. And keep the following tips in mind when experimenting with these products:

+ Choose a commercially prepared sport drink. Commercially prepared fluid replacement drinks contain carbohydrates, sodium and other minerals in amounts that are well absorbed and most likely to be tolerated. Steer clear

Nutrition

10

of recipes for homemade sport drinks, which can be difficult to formulate to the specifications needed to maximize performance.

+ Following the manufacturer's directions when preparing sport drinks from a powdered mix. Add the exact amount of water specified on the label to prepare a drink that provides appropriate amounts of carbohydrates and minerals.

+ Drink small amounts at regular intervals. Consuming large volumes of sport drink in a relatively short period of time can promote bloating and abdominal cramping.

+ Keep it cool. Cool, rather than ice cold fluids are easier to drink in the amounts needed to keep you well hydrated.

Exercise Eating

Pre-Walk Eating

"What should I eat before a walk?" is a common question and one that can haunt you if you have incorrect information. Eating at the wrong time or choosing the wrong kind of foods can produce symptoms like nausea, vomiting and diarrhea, experiences that rarely make for a fun walk!

Eating before activity, or pre-event eating as sport nutritionists refer to it, serves some very important purposes. A sound pre-event meal or snack can

+ enhance endurance
+ prevent hunger and dehydration
+ promote mental alertness

Different people tolerate eating before activity differently, and experimentation is important for finding the exact combination of foods that works best for you. While some walkers can happily down a breakfast of pancakes, sausages and coffee before a walk, others may feel nauseous after eating only a granola bar and a glass of juice. Use your longer training walks to try out different foods and food combinations.

Timing is critical in terms of pre-event eating. Foods need time to be digested in order to serve as a source of energy. Recognizing this, it's important to allow two to four hours between a moderately sized meal and the start of a workout. Smaller snacks or liquid meals can be consumed a little closer to the start of a walk, perhaps as late as one hour before you hit the road.

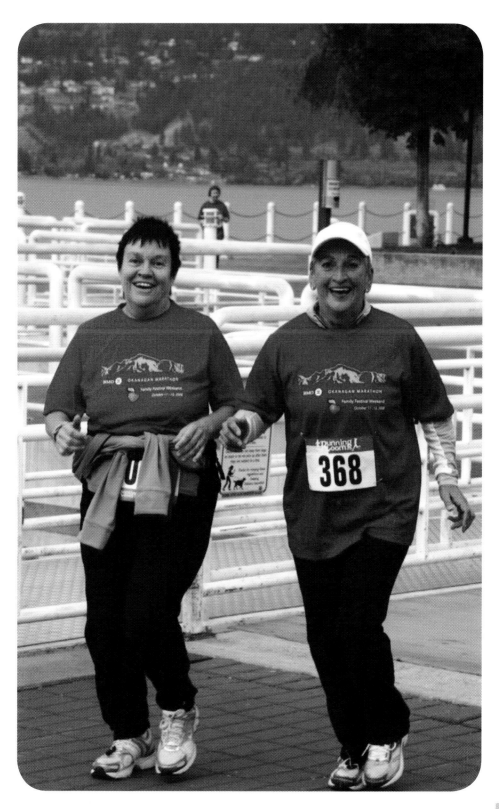

For walkers who enjoy training in the morning, a bedtime snack is critical. A nutritious snack, eaten just before bed, helps to keep blood glucose levels stable. This approach, coupled with a very light snack in the hour prior to a walk, may help you sneak in a bit more sleep before you train.

Some foods offer greater benefits than others as pre-event meal choices. Foods rich in complex carbohydrates, such as breads, pasta, cereals or grains, are broken down quickly to provide the body with a source of glucose and are ideal choices before exercise. Fluids help to hydrate the body and should be part of all pre-event meals.

Some foods are not suitable for inclusion in a pre-event meal. Many people have difficulty tolerating the following kinds of foods, which should be eaten with caution before activity:

+ high sugar foods: honey, regular soft drinks, syrups, candy and table sugars. These foods can cause abdominal cramping and diarrhea.
+ high fiber foods: bran cereals and muffins, legumes (e.g., beans, peas, lentils) and raw vegetables. High fiber foods can produce bloating, gas and diarrhea.
+ high fat or high protein foods: butter, margarine, salad dressings, peanut butter, hamburger, hot dogs, etc. Fat and protein take longer to digest than carbohydrates and are not a good source of quick fuel during exercise.

Examples of Pre-Event Meals and Snacks
Breakfast

250 ml (1 cup) Rice Krispies
250 ml (1 cup) skim milk
1 banana
250–500 ml (1–2 cups) plain, cool water

Snack

1 large cinnamon-raisin bagel
250 ml (1 cup) orange juice
250 ml (1 cup) low fat yogurt
125 ml (½ cup) strawberries

Nutrients During the Walk

Eating during a walk is a strategy designed to keep blood sugar or glucose levels high and promote endurance. Research shows that athletes who consume carbohydrate-rich foods or beverages during prolonged activity benefit from enhanced performance.

A wide variety of foods and drinks are available to provide long distance walkers with the carbohydrates needed to keep blood glucose levels within the normal range. Sport drinks, gels or "Gu," energy bars and even dried fruits are all items that you can use to top up your carbohydrate stores during a walk.

Like the ideal pre-event meal, the definition of a perfect on-the-run snack varies from walker to walker. Keep the following points in mind as you look for foods to eat during activity:

Portability is important. Ideal on-the-run food choices are non-perishable, light-weight and easily contained.

Taste matters! Most walkers will need to take in between 30 g and 60 g of carbohydrate per hour to keep blood glucose levels in the normal range during activity. Translated into food or beverage choices this equals

+ 1 to 2 packages of sport gel
+ 1 sport bar
+ 500 ml (2 cups) of sport drink
+ 60–80 ml (¼–⅜ cup) raisins

Unless you enjoy the taste, taking in the recommended amounts of these foods or beverages will be a challenge.

Experiment. The ability to tolerate sport gels, bars and drinks is highly individual. While some walkers swear by these products, others are unable to tolerate even small amounts. Discover what works best for you by experimenting with a variety of carbohydrate-rich snacks during your long training walks.

10 Nutrition

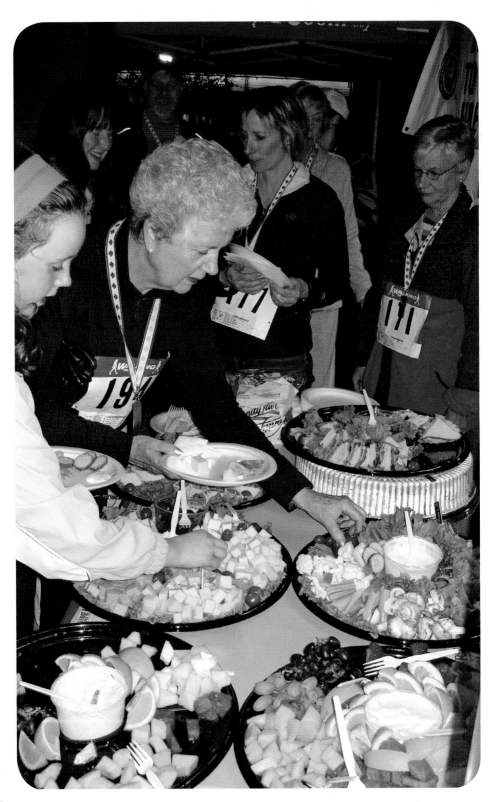

Recovery Eating

Distance walking is intensive, and after a long walk or race the body needs to be refueled. Eating well after exercise can help to speed your recovery and allow you to train at a consistently high level.

Keep the carbs coming! The body is primed to replace its glycogen stores following a long or rigorous bout of exercise. Make the most of this situation by choosing carbohydrate-rich foods and drinks immediately after finishing a workout. Continue to snack on foods like bagels, muffins, cereal and milk, fruits and fruit juices for several hours to fully restore muscle glycogen.

After your exercise continue drinking liquids to combat dehydration by replacing water that was lost from your body during exercise. Once your urine is clear and you are emptying your bladder you can resume to normal hydration.

Loosening Up

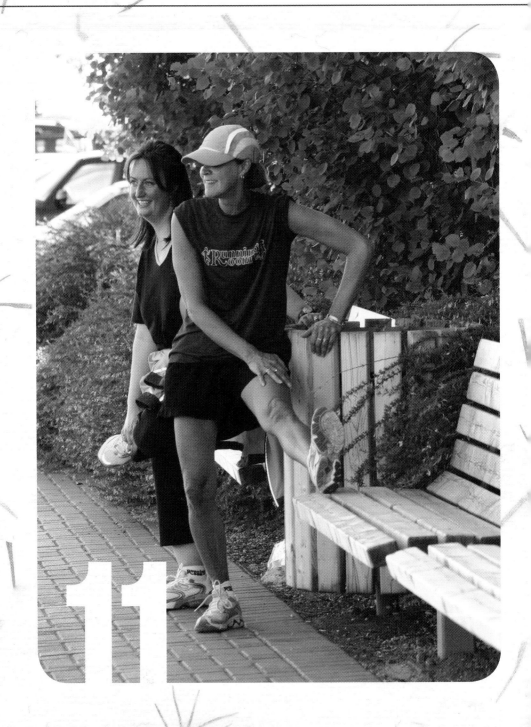

11

Along with aerobic fitness and strength, flexibility is also an important component of total body health and wellness. Simply put, strong flexible muscles perform better and sustain fewer injuries. It has been traditionally believed that performing warm-up exercises that include stretching can help avoid injury during the subsequent activity. Although this belief may not be completely true, a well-planned warm-up, cooldown and stretching regimen are important aspects of every training session.

Warm-Up

The main purpose of a warm-up is to ready the body for the subsequent activity. It assists the heart, lungs and muscles to prepare for the intensity of exercise and to ease the body through the transition between, rest and exercise. There are many forms of warm-up. Calisthenics, stretching and other forms of stationary exercise are popular. The best form of warm-up is doing your planned exercise activity only much more slowly for the first few minutes of the session. For example: Tennis players often warm up playing at the service lines, rather than using the full court. Start your activity on a smaller scale. Start leisurely walking, steady walking and then brisk or even race walking. Be gentle, and progressively increase your intensity through a comfortable zone. How do you know if your warm-up has been long enough? Are you sweating yet? Perspiration is a sure sign that warm-up can end, and your exercise session can begin.

Walking Warm-Up Moves

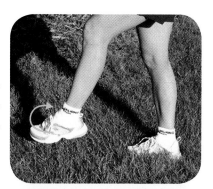

1. Ankle Circles

Stand on one foot and lift the other off the ground. Slowly flex that ankle through its full range of motion, making circles with the toes. Do six to eight in each direction, then switch feet and repeat.

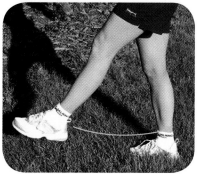

2. Leg Swings

Stand on one leg and swing the other loosely from the hip, front to back. It should be a relaxed, unforced motion like the swinging of a pendulum, and your foot should swing no higher than a foot or so off the ground. Do 15–20 swings on each leg.

Stretching

"Stretching, who me? Well, maybe to get that last chocolate chip cookie on the far side of the table, but not for walking."

A lot of walkers will give you this kind of response when you ask about stretching. The debate on the benefits of stretching has been going on for a while, between athletes who follow a regular routine and athletes who only do the occasional stretch as they blink away the previous night's sleep.

Studies by the sports medicine experts tell us that there is a correlation between injuries and stretching habits. They have found very little difference in injury rates between athletes who stretch on a regular basis and athletes who do not stretch at all, but those who stretch occasionally have the highest incidence of injuries. In looking for a reason for their higher injury rate, they concluded that sporadic stretchers often stretch incorrectly and at the wrong time.

Pure speed has a lot to do with genetics. The rest of us need whatever other advantages we can find. The older I become the more I believe in stretching.

The thing I have found as a coach is that maintaining flexibility is a real factor in maintaining some semblance of speed. Think of the two ways we become faster: a faster leg turnover and a longer stride. As we age, if we do not work at maintaining our flexibility, the stride length of our youth will soon leave us. Even if you are able to maintain your leg turnover, a shorter stride length means slower times.

The repetitive action of walking causes the two major muscle groups, the hamstrings on the back of the high thigh and the quadriceps on the front, to tighten up when put through the relatively limited range of the walking motion. Stretching is integral to maintaining a full range of motion at the ankle, knee and hip.

Stretching is always best done when the muscles are warm. If your preference is to stretch before you work out, then be sure to do a full warm-up first of 10 minutes. On the other hand, stretching can become a part of an extended cool down. If improved flexibility is your goal, then stretching while your muscles are cooling from a training session will give the best results. Never sit down and stretch too soon after your workout. Stretching is only recommended after an appropriate cooldown.

How to Stretch

Stretching should be done slowly without bouncing. Stretch to where you feel a slight, easy stretch (not pain). Hold this feeling for approximately 20 seconds. As you hold the stretch, the feeling of tension should diminish. If it doesn't, ease off slightly into a more comfortable stretch. This easy first stretch readies the tissue for the developmental stretch. After holding the easy stretch, move slightly further into the stretch until you feel mild tension again. This is the developmental stretch, which should be held for 20 to 30 seconds. This feeling of stretch tension should slightly diminish or stay the same. If the tension increases or becomes painful, you are overstretching. Again, ease off to a comfortable stretch.

The developmental stretch reduces the risk of injuries and will safely increase flexibility. Hold the stretch at a tension that feels comfortable to you. The key to stretching is to keep relaxed while you concentrate on the area to be stretched. Your breathing should be regular. Be sure not to hold your breath. Don't worry how far you can stretch in comparison to others—increased personal flexibility is a guaranteed result of a regular stretching program.

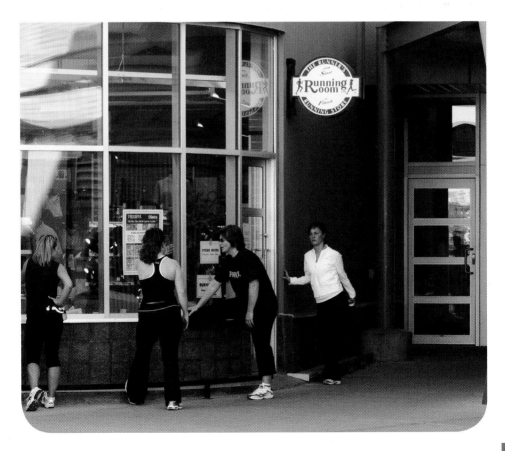

11 Loosening Up

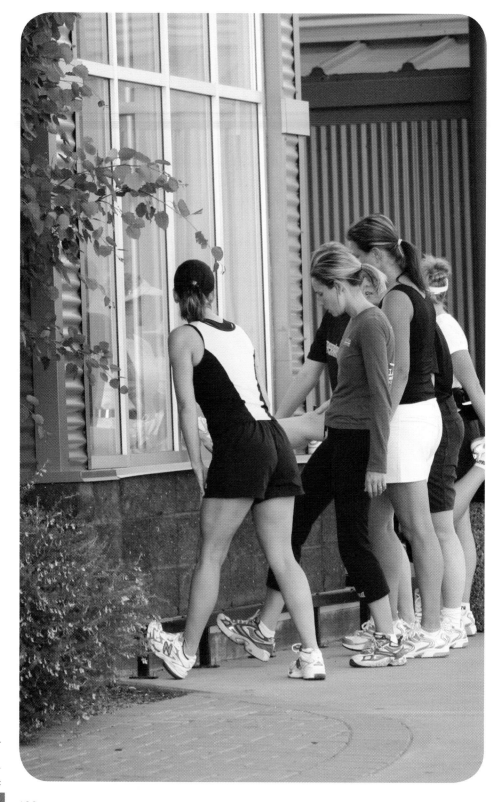

The Stretches

The following are recommended stretches for beginner and novice walkers.

Calf

Stand about 3 ft. (1 m) from a wall, railing or tree with your feet flat on the ground, toes slightly turned inward, heels out and back straight. The forward leg should be bent and the rear leg should be gradually straightened until there is tension in the calf. Finally, bend the straight leg at the knee to work closer to the Achilles tendon.

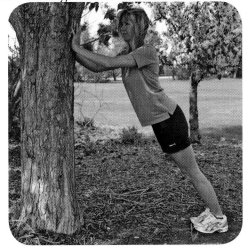

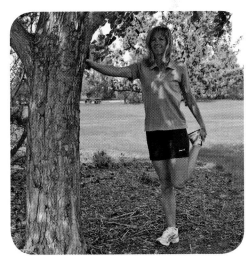

Hamstring

Sit with one leg straight out and your other leg bent behind you. Lean forward and reach for your toes. For an alternate stretch, place one foot on a railing, wall or bench with your knee bent and back straight. Slowly straighten the leg. For an additional stretch, keep your back straight and bend forward.

Quadriceps (also known as "quads")

Place one arm on something handy to balance yourself and use the other hand to pull the foot back when one leg is bent at the knee. The bent knee should touch the other knee. Don't push it forward or pull it back. While this stretch is being executed, the belly button should be pulled up under the rib cage, which is called a pelvic tilt. The tilt protects the back.

11 Loosening Up

Iliotibial Band Stretch

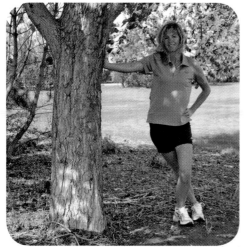

With one leg towards a railing, bench or wall and the other leg slightly bent, cross the leg to be stretched behind the bent leg. Shift your hip towards the wall to stretch the iliotibial band. You should feel the stretch over the hip area.

Buttock Stretch

Sit up straight with one leg straight and the knee of your other leg bent, with the foot of the bent leg on the outside of the straightened leg. Slowly pull the bent leg towards the opposing shoulder. The buttock of the bent leg will be stretched.

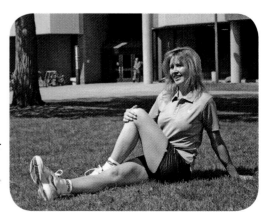

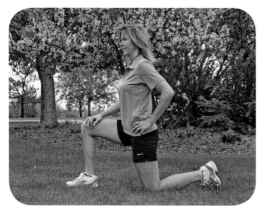

Hip Flexor Stretch

Kneel on one knee and place the other leg forward at a 90-degree stance. Keep the back straight and maintain the pelvic tilt while lunging forward. The rear knee is planted to stretch the hip in front.

Cooldown

The purpose of cooldown is the exact opposite of warm-up. Incorporating a planned cooldown at the end of your exercise session assists the body in the transition from exercise to rest. It allows the heart to adjust to the decreased intensity more slowly and can prevent labored breathing at the end of higher intensity exercise sessions. Blood flow can slow more naturally with a cooldown, which will prevent the pooling of blood in the exercising muscles and thus prevent any dizziness or nausea that can result from suddenly stopping particularly high-intensity exercise. The optimal length of the cooldown period is dependent on the intensity and duration of the prior exercise with the long, more intense sessions requiring an extended cooldown. A cooldown period of 5–10 minutes should suffice for almost every workout. Like the warm-up, the bulk of the activity done during the cooldown should be the same as the exercise session, only slower or on a smaller scale. Finish your walk with a slow stroll or a leisurely walk.

Tips on Stretching

Stretching is always best done when the muscles are warm. If your preference is to stretch before you work out, then be sure to do a full warm-up first (10 minutes). On the other hand, stretching can become a part of an extended cooldown. If improved flexibility is your goal, then stretching while your muscles are cooling from a training session will give the best results. Never sit down and stretch too soon after your workout Stretching is only recommended after an appropriate cooldown.

Walking Sports Medicine

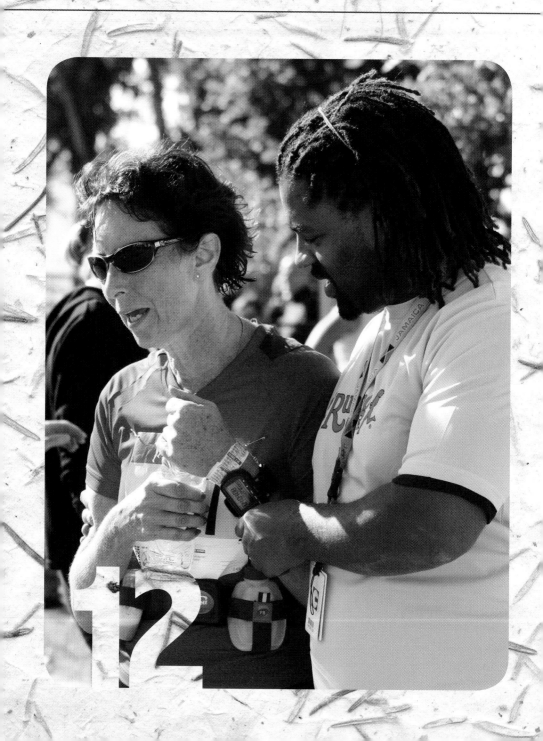

12

Walking Sports Medicine

Most walkers are highly motivated and extremely devoted to their sport. They think that if they don't get their walk in they won't feel quite right. While they are in pursuit of those miles, many forget to listen to their bodies.

Avoiding injury is not impossible if you pay attention to your training techniques and don't try to do too much, too soon. The best way to prevent most athletic injuries is to maintain good muscle strength and flexibility.

Most walking injuries are from overuse, so tune in to your body and listen to what it's telling you. If you're cranky or more impatient than usual, you may need a few days of rest. Other signs of fatigue are a susceptibility to colds or flu, difficulty falling asleep, an inability to sleep well, a higher than usual resting pulse rate or more-than-the-usual aches and pains in the limbs. Remember these wise words: Any pain, no brain.

Common Causes of Injury

+ too many miles, too quickly
+ walking in improper or worn-out shoes
+ insufficient rest, such as walking too hard on "easy" days
+ lack of a good mileage base
+ forcing a walk when you're tired
+ pushing too hard during intervals and tempo walks
+ too much speed training or too many hills

Overuse vs. Traumatic Injuries

Definition

There are two types of injuries that an athlete may encounter: one caused by an acute trauma; the other resulting from overuse.

The Traumatic Injury

The traumatic injury is violent and sudden, such as sprains, lacerations, torn ligaments, pulled muscles or broken bones caused by a fall. These types of injury usually require immediate professional treatment. If the injury causes immediate pain, swelling, inability to use the injured body part or severe pain that does not subside in 30–40 minutes, the injury should be examined by a professional. If the athlete hears or feels a crack, tear or pop and the pain persists, help should be sought.

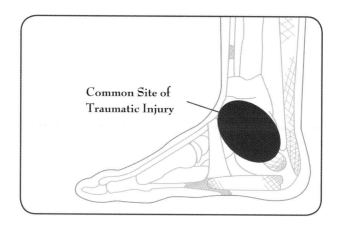

Common Site of
Traumatic Injury

The Overuse Injury

Overuse injuries are more common and develop over a long period of time from mild or low-grade, repeated stress. Overtraining results in overuse injuries. Sometimes this type of injury can be associated with anatomical variation, such as flat or high arches or an abnormally sized or positioned kneecap. The knees (e.g., Iliotibial band syndrome, walker's knee) and Achilles tendon (e.g., tendonitis) are most adversely affected by overtraining.

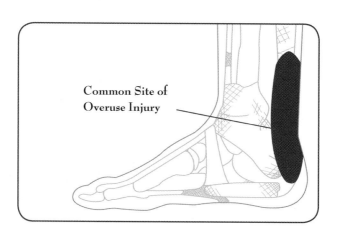

Common Site of
Overuse Injury

Walk Away From Injury

Walking is one of the most injury-free sport activities. However, injuries afflict some of our walking colleagues from time to time.

We should first and foremost marvel at the structural brilliance of our bodies. Walking is made up of many thousands of powerful impacts (1) a repeated action and (2) sudden loading of muscles and connective tissues.

The good news is that in walking the impact forces are reduced by at least 50%. A typical walking injury is actually hard to identify. You certainly don't need to fear a career-ending disaster lurking around the corner, as, for example, baseball pitchers worry about the elbow of their throwing arm or sprinters worry about their hamstrings. Distance runners experience a number of overuse injuries from shin splints, to tendonitis to stress fracture. Walkers aren't really afflicted by a so-called typical injury, but on occasion we can sustain an injury.

The more competitive people are, the higher their work load in duration and intensity. They definitely find themselves reaching for the ice pack now and again. But obviously they don't all injure themselves in the same place. If something gets injured, it's more likely to be a weak link in their training. Walking really can be the perfect, painless route to increased fitness. Listen to your body and adjust your training to your current fitness level

Race Walking

"Doesn't that hurt your hips?" is one of the most common questions race walkers are asked. When people see the typically straight knee of a walker at speed, they are also concerned about race walkers' knees.

Actually, no. The hips and knees don't usually hurt. In the lower part of the body, the reduced impact from walking shelters walkers from all kinds of injury problems. After the low impact, there is another aspect of the sport, which also helps with injury prevention and management. The technique of race walking implies a great deal of mobility. Race walkers are not all naturally flexible. But they all work on the flexibility they have in order to maintain and improve the functional range of movement race walking requires.

Don't be surprised if you notice that the muscles of your upper back are sore after a race or a good workout. This just means that you have been using your shoulders well; the soreness comes from the constant dynamic swing.

One thing that most walkers will agree on: in particular, beginners feel the muscles of the shin working. The requirement to straighten the knee on landing means that the foot is dorsiflexed (pulled back). Much of this soreness is a result of using muscles in a new way. With consistency of training much of this soreness will go away.

Basic Care of Injuries

The pain associated with overuse injuries is usually not severe. It is often ignored by athletes, and it is more difficult to determine whether or not an overuse injury needs professional attention. If the pain persists for more than a few days after you follow basic self-care treatments, such as decreasing the level of activity, applying ice, elevating what is injured, compression, taking aspirin or ibuprofen and stretching, you should seek professional medical help.

Definition

R Rest:
Stop any aggravating activity that could make the injury worse.

I Ice:
The quicker the ice is applied after the injury, the more effective the treatment.

C Compression:
Usually applied using a stretch elastic bandage (tensor type), wrapping towards the heart.

E Elevation:
During and after application of ice, the injured body part should be elevated above the level of the heart.

Regime for R.I.C.E.

+ Do an initial assessment of the injured structure.
+ Within 5–10 minutes following injury, apply ice massage or an ice pack directly to the injured area.
+ An ice pack should be wrapped firmly in place with a wide elastic wrap (be sure to check that circulation isn't impaired).
+ The injured body part should then be elevated well above the level of the heart.
+ Leave the ice pack in place for 15–20 minutes.

- After removing the pack, apply an elastic wrap for compression and continue to elevate the body part.
- Ice should be applied every hour for as many hours as possible during the first 48 hours.
- Use compression at all times, except when sleeping.
- Elevation should continue as often as is practical during this time.

Why Ice?

When you injure yourself, you damage tissue at the site of the injury. Blood vessels inside the tissue break and bleed.

The cold from ice achieves two positive effects. Cold application contracts the broken blood vessels that close quickly and the bleeding stops. Heat on an acute injury can cause the blood vessels to expand.

Blood is also a healing agent. We don't want it spilling into places where it's not supposed to be, but we do need it to flow normally through the tiny blood vessels still intact in the tissue.

Cold brings blood to a cold area in order to warm it—this is why your cheeks and nose go red in winter. The use of ice triggers this protective mechanism. At the same time that the broken blood vessels are being sealed off, the healthy ones are filling with blood. You will notice the redness in the area you are icing after only a few minutes. We are in fact "tricking" the body into thinking that there is a problem with the climate! Good blood flow starts the healing processes almost immediately.

But we can only trick the body for so long because another line of defence is triggered in cases of extreme cold. After trying to warm an area without success, the body's blood supply abandons an area of surface cold and concentrates on the protection of the vital parts of the body. This is what happens in the winter when people suffer frostbite.

So we do not keep the ice on for too long. 15 minutes per hour is plenty. But, for the first 48 hours after an injury, the more hours you can manage with 15 minutes of icing, the better.

How to Ice

1. Your ice pack must allow insulation between the source of cold and the

skin. Without this insulation, the skin can freeze and you have a case of self-inflicted frostbite. Plastic bags do not allow this insulation. Water from the melting ice does! You can apply ice directly onto your skin with no problem, as long as you keep it moving. You can wrap ice cubes in a wet towel or face cloth. But ice in a dry plastic bag on the skin will freeze your skin quite quickly.

Many athletes have Styrofoam cups of water handy in the freezer. They are comfortable to handle and easily peeled back to expose more ice as they melt. They also provide a convenient-sized ice surface.

In general, an ice massage, applied directly onto the skin, but with circular strokes moving over the affected area, is very effective therapy indeed. A cold pack resting on the area may not work as well unless securely held in place.

2. You will feel three stages during your icing. First, of course, your skin feels cold. Second, the injury may actually ache a little, especially if you apply gentle pressure. (The gentle pressure is better than just patting at the area!)

   The third stage will occur after about 10 minutes. The ice will act as a mild anesthetic!

   Try closing you eyes and have another person very gently tap the place that you have iced. You will not be able to feel the tapping.

3. This numbness is the stage you want to reach. For a couple of minutes, you can remove the ice and gently put the injured area through as much range of motion as it can do without pain.

How Long?

While the injury is still acute, ice is what you need. This generally lasts 48 hours and may be longer. If a slight movement reproduces the sharp pain of the original injury, your injury is still acute.

When you feel that the sharp pain has been replaced by a duller ache and a distinct restriction of normal movement, you may move to the next stage in your recovery. If you have visited a therapist, follow the advice you are given. If you are treating the injury yourself, put it through a gentle range of motion and begin as much activity as you can do without causing pain. Pain is absolutely your body's warning signal. Pain indicates that you are causing further damage and delaying your eventual return.

Overtraining

Overtraining is doing too much, too soon. To think that overtraining means you must have increased your workout or be doing high intensity or have increased distance is a misunderstanding of the term. You can overtrain at any level if you are doing too much too soon. It is all relative to your current fitness. Training is the result of the body adapting to stress. The stress must be regular enough and strong enough to stimulate adaptation, but if it is too strong or too frequent, you will break down—you are overtraining. Rest is the phase during which adaptation takes place, and you become stronger. It is just as important as your workout.

Rest is

+ plenty of sleep at night
+ easy days
+ days off
+ alternating activities (e.g., alternating upper-body and lower-body workouts, such as using swimming as a rest from running)

If you do not rest voluntarily, your body will force you to rest—by fatigue, illness, injury, staleness or burnout.

Overtraining is a common cause of poor performance and a common cause of injury. Many personal bests and world records have been set after an injury. This is because an injury is an enforced rest—time for an overtrained body to strengthen and reestablish a balance between stress and adaptation.

Preventing Overtraining

1. Hard Day/Easy Day

Instead of doing the same workout each day, vary your workouts. Therefore, alternate hard and easy days; take days off.

2. The Magic 10s

These may seem conservative, but they are based on sound training principles:

+ Establish a 10-week training base of endurance before doing any competition, speed work or all out efforts.
+ Increase by 10% per week. That means if you're running 30 kilometers a week you should increase to only 33 kilometers the next week.
+ Make only 10% of your weekly workout high intensity (speed work or competition).

3. Morning Resting Pulse Rate

When you wake up, rest in bed for five minutes and then take your pulse. Any day your pulse is up you haven't adapted to or recovered from your previous day. It should be an easy day or a day off.

If you see a drop in performance, your tendency probably is to increase your training. Poor performance is a good indicator of overtraining, so be aware, cut back and apply sound training principles.

Injuries

Achilles Tendonitis

Definition

Achilles tendonitis, one of the more common and difficult injuries to treat in athletes, involves inflammation and degeneration or rupture of the Achilles tendon. The Achilles tendon is located at the back of the heel and inserts into the rear portion of the heel bone. It is surrounded by a vascular sheath that provides the tendon fibers with their blood supply.

Symptoms

The symptoms of this injury tend to come in stages or degrees of severity.

Stage 1

The athlete will experience a burning or prickly pain in the Achilles tendon about one to three inches above the heel bone. This is the result of inflammation of the vascular sheath and may simply be because of shoe counter irritation.

Stage 2

The Achilles tendon actually begins to deteriorate (tendonitis) and the pain becomes a shooting or piercing sensation that occurs during activity, especially when changing direction or running uphill.

Stage 3

The collagen protein fibers in the Achilles tendon weaken to a point that the tendon will snap or rupture, and there will be a great deal of swelling. The main cause of tendon damage is sudden overstretching of tendon fibers. The Achilles tendon must be properly preconditioned to withstand sudden stretches and the strain of body weight during activity. If a chronic tendonitis is ignored and the tendon ruptures, the cells that repair the tendon cannot work quickly enough to heal the damage done by the over-enthusiastic athlete.

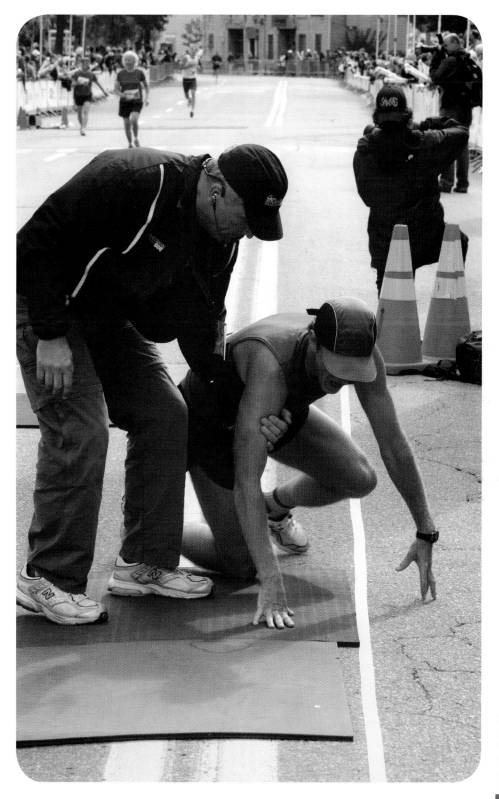

1. The positioning of the tendon in the calf makes it susceptible to walking injuries.

2. Overpronation strains the soleus tendon.

3. Oversupination or high arches strains the gastrocnemius fibers in the calf muscle. Both cause injury high up in the Achilles tendon.

4. Constant rubbing of the back of the shoe against the tendon

5. Improper shoe selection

6. Improper warm-up

7. Direct trauma

8. A sudden dramatic increase in activity or intensity of activity

9. Heel bone deformity

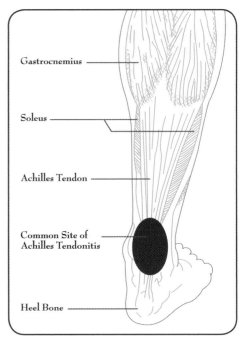

10. A high-mileage, long-term walking program that does not incorporate enough rest

Short-term Treatment

+ decrease mileage and intensity for 7–10 days; never walk through pain
+ avoid hills and sped during recovery; both can exacerbate
+ ice treatment after walking
+ flexibility program concentrating on the soleus and gastrocnemius, including stretching and heel lifts
+ Aspirin or ibuprofen to reduce inflammation
+ orthotic devices or proper shoe selection

If the injury persists for more than two weeks, it is recommended that the athlete see a physician.

Long-term Treatment

+ continuous flexibility program

- orthotic devices
- professional treatment by a physician may be required

For overall prevention of injury, all athletes should be aware of shoe deterioration and purchase shoes designed to correct any stride problems, such as overpronation or oversupination.

Iliotibial Band Syndrome

Definition

Iliotibial band syndrome is one of the leading causes of lateral knee pain in runners. The iliotibial band is a superficial thickening of tissue on the outside of the thigh, extending from the outside of the pelvis, over the hip and knee, and inserting just below the knee. The band is crucial to stabilizing the knee during running, moving from behind the femur to the front of it during the gait cycle. The continual rubbing of the band over the bone, combined with the repeated flexion and extension of the knee during running may cause the area to become inflamed or the band itself may become irritated.

Symptoms

The symptoms range from a stinging sensation just above the knee joint on the outside of the knee or along the entire length of the iliotibial band to swelling or thickening of the tissue at the point where the band moves over the femur. The pain may not occur immediately, but it will worsen during activity when the foot strikes the ground if you overstride or walk downhill. It may persist afterward. A single workout of excessive distance or a rapid increase in weekly distance can aggravate the condition.

Causes of Injury

- Iliotibial band syndrome is the result of both poor training habits and anatomical abnormalities.
- Walking on a banked surface, such as the shoulder of a road or an indoor track, causes the downhill leg to bend slightly inward and causes extreme stretching of the band against the femur.
- You have an inadequate warm-up or cooldown.
- Walking excessive distances or increasing mileage too quickly can aggravate or cause injury.
- You have anatomical abnormalities, such as bowlegs or tightness about the iliotibial band.

To treat functional problems resulting from poor training

+ decrease distance
+ ice knee after activity
+ alternate walking direction on a pitched surface
+ use a lateral sole wedge to lessen pressure on the knee
+ stretch to tolerance

To treat structural abnormalities, such as a natural tightness in the band

+ stretch, especially before working out, to make the band more flexible and less susceptible to injury
+ in extreme cases, surgery to relieve tightness in the band
+ both structural and functional problems need to be considered when treating iliotibial band syndrome

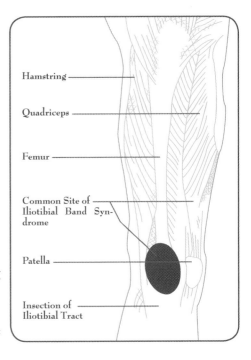

Hamstring

Quadriceps

Femur

Common Site of Iliotibial Band Syndrome

Patella

Insection of Iliotibial Tract

Plantar Fasciitis

Plantar fasciitis is a persistent pain located on the plantar aspect (bottom) of the heel and the medial aspect (inside) of the foot. The plantar fascia is a fibrous, tendon-like structure that extends the entire length of the bottom of the foot, beginning at the heel bone and extending to the base of the toes. During excessive activity, the plantar fascia can become irritated and inflamed and may even tear if the area is subjected to repetitive stress. Heel contact during the gait cycle exposes a specific area to this stress. This area is known as the medial plantar aspect of the heel, where the plantar fascia attaches to the heel bone. The pain resulting from this injury is most noticeable in the morning when the first few steps are taken and subsides with prolonged walking. Likewise, during athletic activity the pain will occur in the beginning of the exercise routine and subsides as activity continues.

+ Plantar fasciitis is more common in athletes who have a high-arch, rigid type of foot or a flat, pronated foot. In motion, the plantar fascia experiences continuous stress and excessive pulling, which results in inflammation and pain.

- A high-arch foot has a tight band-like plantar fascia that is rigid during the gait cycle.
- The plantar fascia is stretched by excessive motion in the pronated foot.
- Improper shoe selection can be a cause of the injury; foot and gait type must be considered.
- Stiff-soled shoes can cause stretching of the plantar fascia.
- Overworn shoes allow the foot to pronate more extensively and can result in an injury to the plantar fascia.
- The most common cause is a sudden increase in the amount or intensity of activity within a short period of time.

Short-term Treatment

In determining the proper treatment for plantar fasciitis it is important that the athlete knows and eliminates the causative factors of the injury. A complete medical history analysis, pedal examination, gait analysis and X-rays to check for a heel spur are recommended. Also you can do the following:

- ice application and strapping
- complete rest or a reduction in the intensity of exercise
- physical therapy involving whirlpool and ultrasound
- anti-inflammatory medication, such as pills, liquid penetrating rubs or cortisone injections, to alleviate severe pain in acute cases. These are considered only as a last resort in chronic cases only.

Long-term Treatment

In cases that are persistent, orthotic devices help correct biomechanical problems and alleviate stress and strain on the plantar fascia.

- High arches require softer orthotic devices for shock absorption.
- Flattened arches require a more rigid orthotic to control pronation.
- Plantar fascia and calf muscle stretching exercises can prevent recurrence.

Most patients respond to these forms of treatment; only a very small percentage of patients require surgery.

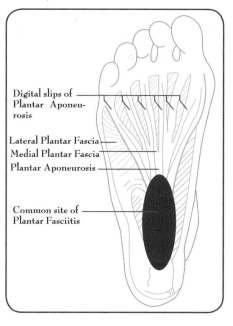

Digital slips of Plantar Aponeurosis

Lateral Plantar Fascia
Medial Plantar Fascia
Plantar Aponeurosis

Common site of Plantar Fasciitis

Stress Fractures

Stress fractures are tiny, incomplete breaks or cracks in a normal bone caused by repeated trauma or pounding. One of the most misdiagnosed of athletic injuries, stress fractures can happen after a short period of stress, but more commonly after a longer period of continued trauma. When the bone cells cannot rebuild as fast as the repetitive trauma damages them and the bone can take no more stress, the crack occurs. Stress fractures can occur in both the upper and lower body, but they are most common in the foot.

Symptoms

The pain related to a stress fracture begins gradually and intensifies with continued activity. Pain is not always present as an early warning, or it is often ignored by the athlete. Swelling and tenderness may also affect the area. One of a physician's best methods in determining a stress fracture is if pain is felt when pressure is applied from above and below. X-rays of the injured site should be taken, though the fracture may not show up for the first 5–10 days after the injury. When stress fractures are ignored, the results can be serious. Complete breaks in the bone, especially in the hip area, may necessitate surgery or prolonged disability.

Causes of Injury

+ switching to a harder running surface
+ rapid increase of speed or distance
+ returning to intense activity after a layoff
+ inadequate rest and excessive stress
+ a change in footwear without proper adjustment period
+ improper shoe selection to accommodate foot type

Most athletes who incur stress fractures are in good physical condition and lack previous systemic ailments that may predispose them to the injury.

Short-term Treatment

+ discontinue the injurious activity immediately
+ rest
+ ice
+ elevation

If pain and swelling do not subside after a few days of self-prescribed care, and if athletic as well as normal activities become difficult, professional help should be sought.

- non impact aerobic activity, such as swimming, rowing, cross-country skiing, or bicycling, to maintain cardiovascular fitness

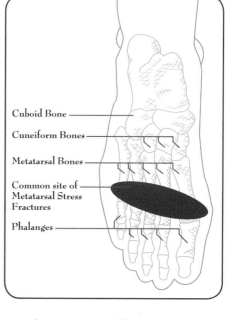

Cuboid Bone

Cuneiform Bones

Metatarsal Bones

Common site of Metatarsal Stress Fractures

Phalanges

- a cast may be used in tibial (lower leg) stress fractures; metatarsal (foot) stress fractures may require casting for four to six weeks because these bones are more difficult to immobilize
- a heel cup or special protective padding for heel fractures
- crutches to relieve the pressure and weight from the leg
- oral nonsteroidal anti-inflammatory medications to alleviate pain and swelling

The return to athletic activity should be delayed for as long as possible—from four to eight weeks—depending on the location and severity of the injury. Though the pain may subside after the second week of treatment, returning to a normal exercise routine can delay healing and can cause permanent damage.

Shin Splints
Definition

The lower leg pain resulting from shin splints is caused by very small tears in the leg muscles at their point of attachment to the shin. There are two types:

- Anterior shin splints occur in the front portion of the shin bone (tibia).
- Posterior shin splints occur on the inside (medial) part of the leg along the tibia.
- Anterior shin splints are due to muscle imbalances, insufficient shock absorption or toe running. Excessive pronation contributes to both anterior and posterior shin splints.

Symptoms

The pain may begin as a dull aching sensation after running. The aching may become more intense, during walking, if ignored. Tender areas are often felt as one or more small bumps along either side of the shin bone.

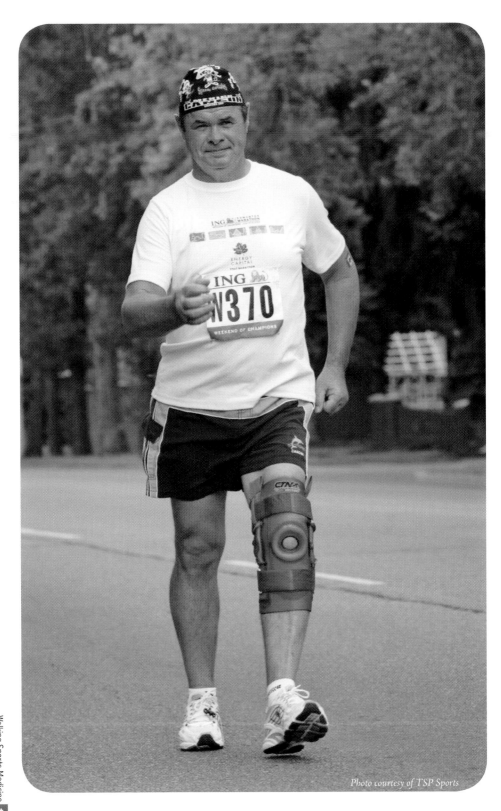

+ Tightness in the posterior muscles, which propel the body forward, places additional strain on the muscles in the front part of the lower leg, which work to lift the foot upward and also prepare the foot to strike the walking surface.

+ Hard surface walking and worn or improper shoes will increase the stress on the anterior leg muscles. Softer surfaces and shoe cushioning materials absorb more shock and less is transferred to the shins.

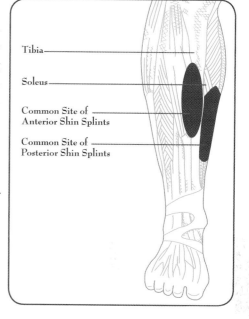

Tibia

Soleus

Common Site of Anterior Shin Splints

Common Site of Posterior Shin Splints

+ The lower leg muscles suffer a tremendous amount of stress when a walker lands only on the balls of the feet (toe walking), without the normal heel contact.

+ The muscles of the foot and leg overwork in an attempt to stabilize the pronated foot and the repeated stress can cause the muscles to tear where they attach to the tibia.

+ You too rapidly increase speed or distance.

Short-term Treatment

+ Aspirin or ibuprofen to reduce inflammation and relieve pain
+ ice immediately after walking, never before
+ reduce distance and intensity for 7–10 days; never walk through pain
+ avoid hills and hard walking surfaces
+ a varus wedge to support the inside of the foot and reduce the amount of pronation
+ gentle stretching of the posterior leg and thigh muscles

Self-enforced treatment of shin splints, as with most overuse injuries, is successful in most cases.

Long-term Treatment

Persistent problems may warrant a visit to a sports medicine specialist who may prescribe the following treatments:

+ strengthening and flexibility programs to correct muscle imbalance; these

exercises should only be done in the absence of pain
+ orthotic devices
+ anti-inflammatory medications
+ physical therapy involving ice, massage, ultrasound, electro-stimuli and heat to reduce inflammation and pain

The best means of prevention of serious athletic injuries is to maintain good muscle strength and flexibility.

Walker's Knee Pain

Definition

Chondromalacia patella, or walker's knee pain, occurs when repeated stress on the knee causes inflammation and a gradual softening of the cartilage under the kneecap (patella). The inflammation of the cartilage prevents the kneecap from gliding smoothly over the end of the thigh bone (femur) therefore causing pain and swelling of the knee. The underside of the kneecap should be smooth and move within the femoral groove (a groove on the thigh bone). If the kneecap is pulled sideways, it becomes rough like sandpaper and the symptoms appear.

Symptoms

Walker's knee is typically associated with a pain that increases gradually over a period of time, often a year or longer, until it is severe enough that the athlete seeks medical attention. Symptoms usually occur beneath or on both sides of the kneecap. Pain may be intensified with activities such as a short walk, squatting or jumping. Stiffness may occur simply from prolonged sitting or descending stairs.

Causes of Injury

+ Overpronation causes the lower leg to rotate inward because of the unstable pronated foot. The kneecap moves in an abnormal side-to-side motion instead of gliding within the normal track of the femoral groove on the thigh bone.
+ Weak quadriceps may contribute to injury because the thigh muscles normally aid in proper tracking of the kneecap.
+ You have muscle imbalance.
+ You have direct or repeated trauma.
+ You have an untreated ligament injury.
+ Some athletes may experience pain in one knee if they continually walk along the same side of the road. The tilt in the road accentuates the pronation of the foot, thus resulting in the abnormal tracking of the knee.

+ You have a history of trauma.

Short-term Treatment

+ Decrease activity and consider swimming. When recovering, avoid any exercise that puts weight on a bent knee.
+ Rest if the knee is painful and swollen.
+ Do an ice treatment for 15 minutes twice daily after the activity to reduce pain and inflammation.
+ Use Aspirin or ibuprofen. Or consult your physician about more sophisticated and effective anti-inflammatory medication.

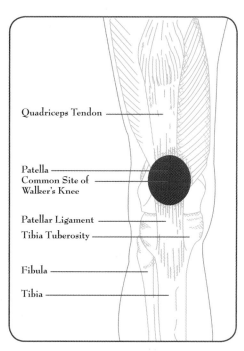

Quadriceps Tendon

Patella
Common Site of
Walker's Knee

Patellar Ligament
Tibia Tuberosity

Fibula

Tibia

Long-term Treatment

+ Go to physiotherapy. Learn stretching and strengthening exercises for the quadriceps, hamstrings and calves.
+ Use orthotic devices to correct abnormal foot mechanics.
+ Once the causes are determined and the appropriate steps have been taken to treat the condition, walker's knee should not keep the athlete from activity.

Cross Training &
Core Strengthening

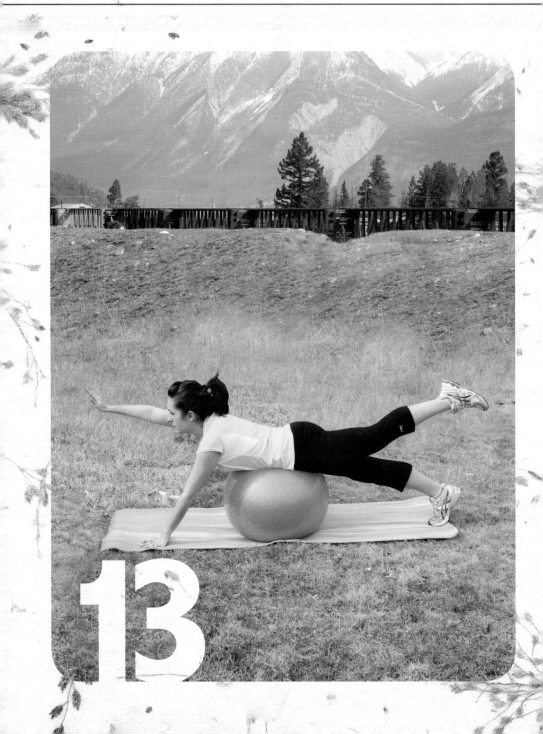

13

Introduction

In this section we will introduce alternative aerobic and strengthening activities to complement your walking program. Both the body and the mind need change—something different from the core training program to add balance and variety. Sticking to one activity, in this case walking, can result in the activity getting a bit stale and also allows for repetitive training injuries to start creeping up on you. The best balance for this is to add in a variety of alternative workouts that will complement your walking training programs and also add strengthening programs to increase your overall core fitness. These activities will serve to make you a better walker, a fitter walker and a less injured walker.

In this chapter we will highlight water workouts and core strength workouts, which include ball exercises, body weight exercises and resistance training exercises.

Water Workouts

Today's athletes are always looking for ways to train more intelligently and improve recovery for hard effort days or injury. Water walking is a great choice, giving many of the same benefits as dry land walking with a lower impact.

Many athletes discovered the benefits of water walking as a recovery from injury. It is possible to walk in the water when an injury does not allow dry land walking. Check with your doctor if you are not sure whether your particular injury allows you to walk in the water.

Once healed, these same athletes often continue water walking, incorporating it into their regular schedule. Water walking can be used to work on technique and range of motion. You can do gentle aerobic walks or high-quality workouts. If you are involved in a program of racing, you can walk in the water at a high effort race pace before or after you would do so on dry land. In the dark, cold days of winter, a pool walk can be a great way for your group to meet socially for a pleasantly warm and well-lit training session.

How to Walk in the Water

Only a very few people are truly uncomfortable in water. Most people can water walk even if they cannot swim.

You need a pool deep enough so that you do not touch the bottom when your

13 Cross Training & Core Strengthening

head and neck are out of the water. A flotation device will give you an added feeling of security. More importantly, it will assist in maintaining a good posture. I recommend the Aqua Jogger.

Above all, the idea is to remember that you are walking. The resistance of the water will slow your walking action somewhat, but in your mind's eye, you should always "see" yourself walking on dry land. The motion may actually be a little slower, much like you are in a movie walking in slow, moderately exaggerated form.

Common Errors and Ways to Improve

1. Leaning far forward, bending at the waist and letting your behind drift up towards the surface. You wouldn't walk that way, so straighten up and push your hips forward. If you can't "feel" this position, practice as follows: Go to the side of the pool and face the side, hanging on with both hands. Drop your feet directly underneath you in the water. Hang there for a while so that you feel the position. Now, turn through 90 degrees and hang on with one hand only. Practice the walking action gently with your legs and your other hand. Keep your feet directly underneath you. When you're comfortable, let go and walk on your own. But don't forget the feeling and range of motion of your legs and arms. Rehearse it any time you need to remind yourself.

2. Too slow and wide a leg action. Remember, you are walking. Some athletes think that the action is done slowly and are surprised at the proper feeling. They report that it's like riding a very small bike. You should only extend the range of motion of your stride when you have a quick rhythm with small strides.

3. Elbows coming up to the side, sometimes reaching the surface. Focus on keeping your arms under the water, driving forward and back from the shoulder. Driving the elbow back creates an action for which there is a reaction. The motion of your arms moving back results in your core body moving forward. Your arms move just as they would in a walking workout.

What You May Feel

1. When you walk in the water, you are learning a new skill and improving your walking form. Some time is needed to acquire the skill. Start by

practicing the action for no more than 30 seconds. It is quite natural to feel awkward at first, but your coordination will improve with practice. Practice, briefly rest and resume your practice. This is the way in which you learn a new skill and develop your running form.

2. Water walking leaves you fatigued, but not sore. The feeling may be deceptive: you're fine in the water, but there is a slight heaviness in your muscles when you get out. Many athletes comment they need a nap after these sessions.

3. Have a drink before you get into the pool and keep a water bottle on the deck and sip every 10 minutes. You still sweat and dehydrate, even though you are immersed in water. Some people are prone to cramping calf muscles after some time in the pool. These muscles are actually working hard against the water resistance. Good hydration helps prevent cramping.

Water Walking Workouts

You can do long and gentle workouts in the water as well as workouts of higher intensity. A great way to recover from a race or a long walk is a 45-minute water walk. Some athletes walk in the water for up to two hours as a substitute for a long walk.

Interval workouts are also possible. The support provided by the water means that rest recoveries can be greatly reduced. Rest recoveries of 60 seconds are considered long, 30 seconds is usual and 15–20 seconds is quite possible. The combinations are limited by your imagination. The example below gives you 16 minutes of high-intensity work. With a warm-up and cooldown of 10 minutes each, the total session time is 45 minutes. The period of high-intensity walking is much longer than you would do on dry land, and the risk of injury is minimal.

Warm up with four intervals of 15 seconds hard with 15 seconds rest between. Than start a ladder:

4 x 30 seconds	(20 sec recovery)
4 x 45 seconds	(30 sec recovery)
4 x 60 seconds	(30 sec recovery)
4 x 45 seconds	(30 sec recovery)
4 x 15 seconds	(20 sec recovery)

Some groups have developed effective water training exercise routines in the shallow end of the pool as well. These are useful for general fitness, and for specific form drills for advanced athletes in many events who need to improve and focus on correct movements.

Deep water walking is the activity of choice for athletes in aerobic activities. Whether it is used as a method of rehabilitation during and after an injury, or a cross training activity to provide variety to an overall program, your water walking places you in the company of many of the country's leading athletes who use water walking or running as an integral part of their long-term training.

Good Water Walking Form

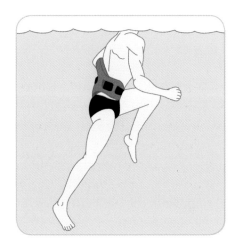

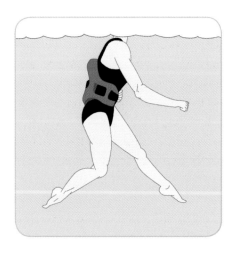

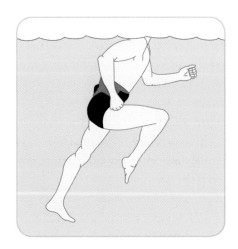

Building Core Strength

Cross training works best when more than one aerobic activity is combined throughout the week with core strength training using weights or some other form of strength exercise. This is a form of cross training that will really complement your aerobic work.

Walking success is a combination of your cardiovascular system (heart, lungs and blood) and your muscles. The energy you are producing is transferred to the ground by your muscles. This transfer moves you forward. The stronger your muscles are, the more effective your walking form.

Walkers do not have to spend the amount of time in the gym that participants in power/speed events often do. Moderate core strength training twice a week will have a significant effect on your aerobic activity. Your muscles will be stronger; so will your connective tissues, resulting in more stable and balanced joints. This applies regardless of gender and it applies to adults of all ages.

As an aerobic athlete, you may not be familiar with core strength exercise, weight room equipment and procedures. The weight room in a modern fitness center is a bright, airy place filled with safe, interesting equipment. It is also staffed by trainers who are more than happy to help you with a program designed to complement your chosen aerobic activity. Do not be intimidated by the fitness room—with a little knowledge and some practice you will soon discover the benefits of strength training. You will feel better, stand taller, experience less injuries and be able to walk longer and faster.

Core Exercises on the Ball

Exercise ball workouts have become very popular over the last few years. They are a great way to lose weight and get in shape and are inexpensive. You do not need to go to a gym because the exercise ball is convenient and easy to use at home. A primary benefit of exercising with an exercise ball is that the body responds to the instability of the ball to remain balanced, engaging many more muscles to do so. These exercises on the ball help strengthen core muscles. They also improve balance and overall coordination. Those muscles become stronger over time to keep balance.

We will demonstrate a few great exercise ball techniques that will soon become a core part of your fitness program. Most of these moves are not advanced exercises that require previous experience with an exercise ball, so enjoy this great training technique.

The Benefits of Using an Exercise Ball

As you will learn later in this chapter, strength training boosts your metabolism by building lean muscle mass. With an exercise ball and a little space, you can build muscle and increase your metabolism with a full-body workout. You will enjoy the following benefits:

- improved balance
- better coordination
- increased flexibility
- enhanced muscle tone
- stronger core

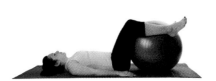

figure 1-a

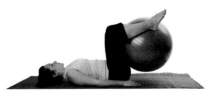

figure 1-b

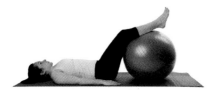

figure 2-a

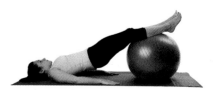

figure 2-b

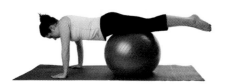

figure 3-a

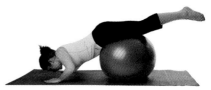

figure 3-b

Ten Simple Exercises

Before you begin the workout, warm up with five minutes of walking or stretching that gets your heart pumping.

1. Inner-Thigh Crunch

Targets: inner thighs and abdominals

Lie on your back with your knees bent at 90 degrees and your shins parallel to the floor. Place the ball between your knees and squeeze your legs together to hold it there. If you have lower-back pain, place your hands under the small of your back for support. (figure 1-a)

Keeping your lower back on the floor, inhale and lift your heels (with your knees still bent) toward the ceiling. Exhale and lower your feet and legs back to the starting position. (figure 1-b)

Repeat 10 times.

2. Bridge

Targets: back of thighs, buttocks and abdominals

Lie on your back with your legs extended, feet hip width apart, and calves and ankles resting on the ball. (figure 2-a)

Exhale, engage your abdominal muscles, and lift your butt toward the ceiling, taking care not to arch your back. Hold for two to five seconds, and then slowly lower yourself back to the starting position. (figure 2-b)

Make this move more difficult by moving the ball closer to your ankles or easier by resting it under your knees. Try for 10 repetitions.

Once you've mastered this move, add a kick. With your butt lifted, shift your weight to your right leg and raise your left leg 90 degrees, keeping your leg straight. Focus on squeezing the thigh and butt muscles in your right leg.

Repeat on the other side for a total of 10 repetitions.

3. Push-Up

Targets: chest, triceps, abdominals, shoulders and back

Lie on the ball on your stomach. Carefully walk your hands forward on the floor until the ball is centered on your thighs. Extend your legs and hold your body in a straight line. (figure 3-a)

Inhale, bend your elbows and lower your chest to the floor. (figure 3-b)

Exhale and push back up to the plank position. Keep your back flat. If this is too difficult, perform the move while resting on your knees.

Repeat as many times as you can, eventually working up to 10 repetitions.

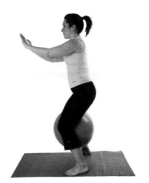

figure 4-a

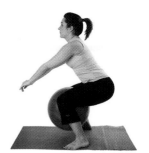

figure 4-b

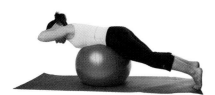

figure 5-a

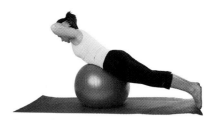

figure 5-b

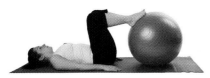

figure 6-a

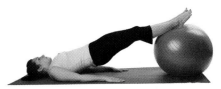

figure 6-b

4. Standing Ball Squeeze

Targets: abdominals, hips, lower back and inner thighs

Stand upright with your hands on a wall or chair for balance. Place the ball between your legs. (figure 4-a)

Kneel forward in a squatting position so your knees hug the ball. Let go of the wall (or chair) and hold your body in a stable stance. This move challenges almost all of your muscles as they work to keep you balanced and steady. (figure 4-b)

Hold the position as long as you can, with a goal of 30 seconds.

This exercise is more difficult with a big ball and easier with a smaller one. This move works your entire body, but you'll feel it most in your inner thighs.

5. Back Extension

Targets: back and shoulders

Facing away from a wall, kneel with the ball in front of you and place your hands behind your head with your elbows bent. Lean forward onto the ball, holding your feet against the wall for stability. Your chest should rest across the top of the ball. (figure 5-a)

Exhale and lift your chest up, stopping when your back is extended in a straight line. Squeeze your shoulder blades together and hold your back tight. Inhale and slowly lower back to the starting position. (figure 5-b)

Repeat 10 times.

Bump up the difficulty by extending your arms straight in a Superman position while you perform the exercise.

6. Hamstring Curl

Targets: abdominals and back of thighs

Lie on your back with your knees bent and your heels resting on the ball. (figure 6-a)

Lift your butt, inhale, and use your feet to push the ball away from you until your legs are straight. (figure 6-b)

Exhale and pull the ball back to the starting position. After 10 repetitions, exhale, tuck your abdominals, and roll back down onto your back.

Once this move becomes easy, take it up a notch by performing the move one leg at a time. In the starting position, shift your weight to your right leg and lift your left leg off the ball. Do the exercise as before, moving the ball with your right leg

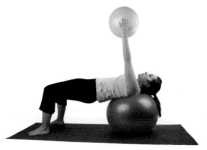

figure 8-a

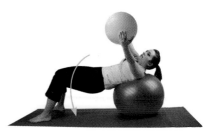

figure 8-b

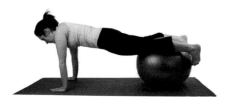

figure 7-a

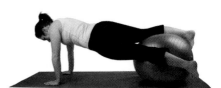

figure 7-b

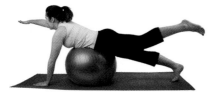

figure 9-a

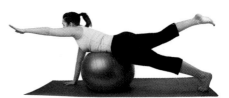

figure 9-b

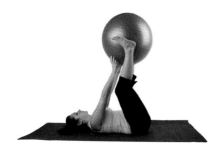

figure 10-a

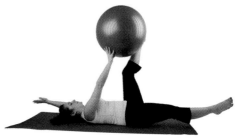

figure 10-b

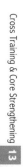

while your left leg hovers above the ball.
After 10 repetitions, switch legs.

7. Ball Rotation (figure 7-a, b)

Targets: abdominals and backs of thighs and shoulders
Lie with the ball under your shoulders and lower back. Extend your arms straight up over your chest, with the palms together. Hold your body in a straight line from hips to knees. Tightening your glutes and abs, slowly twist your body to the left, sweeping your arms parallel to the floor, then back up, repeating on the other side. Try not to collapse the body or roll too far, but really use your abs. Repeat 10 times.

8. Ball Twist (figure 8-a, b)

Targets: abdominals, inner thighs and shoulders
Get into a pushup position with the feet on either side of the ball (turning your ankles so that you are hugging the ball). Hold your body in a straight line with your abs pulled in, hips straight and hands directly under your shoulders. Slowly twist the ball to the right while trying to keep your shoulders level, then to the left. Don't sag in the middle. Repeat 10 times.

9. Opposite Limb Extension (figure 9-a, b)

Targets: lower back, buttocks and hamstrings
Lie with your stomach on the ball and stabilize yourself with your toes and hands. While looking down at the floor, extend your left arm and your right leg simultaneously, hold for two seconds, and return to the starting position. Repeat with the opposite arm and leg combination. Repeat 10 times.

10. The Beetle (figure 10-a, b)

Targets: abdominals, lower back, buttocks, hamstrings and shoulders
Lie down on a matt with the legs and arms straight up. Place the ball between the feet and hands while squeezing to keep the ball in place. Lower your left arm and your right leg simultaneously towards the floor. Keep the knees bent and limit how far you lower the arms and legs. Do not touch the floor. Bring your arm and leg back up, returning to the starting position. Repeat and with the opposite arm and leg combination. Repeat 10 times.

Resistance Training

Basic Principles

What is resistance training?

Resistance training, sometimes called weight training or strength training, is a "specialized method of conditioning designed to increase muscle strength, muscle endurance and muscle power," according to the American Sports Medicine Institute (ASMI). Resistance training can be done in several ways: with resistance machines, free-weights (dumbbells and barbells), rubber tubing or your own body weight (e.g., push-ups, squats or abdominal crunches). The goal of resistance training, the ASMI says, is to "gradually and progressively overload the musculoskeletal system so it gets stronger." Research shows that regular resistance training will strengthen and tone muscles and increase bone mass.

Body Weight Strength Exercises

Question:

Is it necessary to use weights with resistance exercises? I don't have any access to equipment. Can I just do exercises at home without weights?

Answer:

Yes, your own body can function as strength equipment. You can lift it, lower it, curl it, twist it and bend it in all sorts of ways that are designed to increase your strength. I'm talking leg lifts, push-ups, squats, pull-ups. When you move your body weight, you're fighting gravity and that can be a considerable fight.

The advantages of using your body as a weight machine: no cost, no storage and easy to do if your travel a lot.

Body Weight Strength Exercises

Introduction

While stretching helps reduce the risk of injury by keeping muscles and tendons from becoming rigid and inflexible, strengthening helps to prevent injury by keeping weak muscles from being overpowered by stronger ones. The three basic opposing muscle groups for training include:

+ abdominal vs. lower back
+ quadriceps vs. hamstrings
+ anterior shin muscle (front of leg, below knee) vs. calf/Achilles

Also important is the iliotibial band, which is vital in stabilizing the lower leg during walking. It is the most commonly inflamed structure on the outside of the knee, and in walkers it is a frequent cause of pain and soreness at the outer hip.

The hamstring is vulnerable to strains if it is overpowered by the quadriceps. The hamstring therefore demands both stretching and strengthening in a total conditioning program. While your quadriceps are often strong already, they can also benefit from further strengthening to help prevent overuse problems that involve the kneecap.

Strengthening exercises should be done after walking, rather than before. For maximum benefit it is recommended that you follow this routine three to four times per week.

Ankle Exercises

Your ankle acts as a powerful lever during walking. Walkers develop powerful walking-specific muscles, but sometimes neglect the development of improved coordination. Spend some time on the following two drills and not only will they help improve your walking but they may help prevent an injury.

The Flamingo (figure 11-a, 11-b)

Start by balancing on one leg for 30 seconds without touching down with the other leg. When this balance becomes easy, try it with your eyes closed. You will notice it's much harder to hold a balanced position without visual cues. After mastering the blind flamingo, try bending your raised leg slightly at the knee and then do some toe raises.

Cross Training & Core Strengthening

13

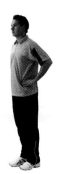 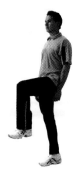

figure 11-a   figure 11-b

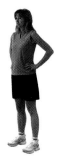 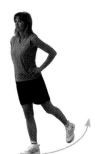 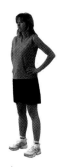 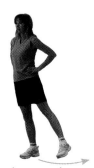

figure 12-a   figure 12-b   figure 12-c   figure 12-d

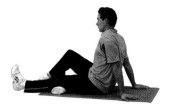 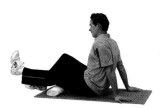

figure 13-a   figure 13-b

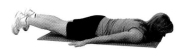 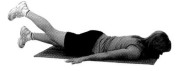

figure 14-a   figure 14-b

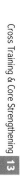

Over the years I have spent a fair amount of time in airport lineups, and I have found the flamingo to be the ideal exercise. You will get some interesting looks, and be careful not to lose your place in the line while your eyes are closed.

Balance Kicks (figure 12-a, 12-d)

This drill can be done on a flat surface, or to increase the complexity try it on a re-bounder. Stand on one leg, kick your other leg back, balance and hold for 20–30 seconds. Switch legs and repeat. Repeat the exercise with kicks out to the side and in front of you. These positions will seem awkward when you first try them, but over time, as your balance improves, they will become more fluid.

Lower Leg Strengthening

Quadriceps (figure 13-a, 13-b)

Terminal Extensions
Sit down. Bend one leg and extend the other. Place a rolled towel under the knee of the extended leg. Lean back on your elbows. Straighten the extended leg and lift it 2 inches above the towel. Hold for three seconds. Complete 10 repetitions; then repeat with the other leg.

Hamstrings (figure 14-a, 14-b)

Hip Extensions
Lie on your stomach with your legs extended. Raise one leg about 6 inches, keeping your knee straight. Hold for three seconds. Keep the hip muscles relaxed. Complete 10 repetitions; then repeat with the other leg.

Tibialis Anterior (figure 15-a, 15-b)

Ankle up-and-down
Sit down with your legs extended and together. Place a loop of Thera-Band around your feet. Bend one knee and pull that foot towards your head. Hold for three seconds. Complete 10 repetitions; then repeat with the other leg. This exercise helps prevent shin splints.

Post Tibialis (figure 16-a, 16-b)

Ankle Eversion
Sit down with your legs extended and together. Place a Thera-Band loop around your feet and hold. Point your toes down and out.

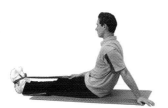

figure 15-a

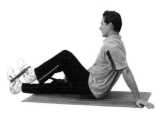

figure 15-b

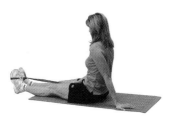

figure 16-a

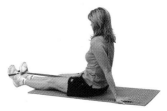

figure 16-b

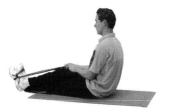

figure 17-a

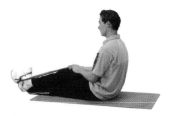

figure 17-b

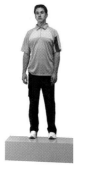

figure 18-a

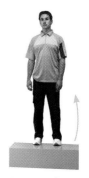

figure 18-b

Ankle Inversion

Sit down with your legs extended and crossed. Place a Thera-Band loop around your feet and hold. Point your toes down and out.

Lower Body Strength Training

Foot and Leg Exercise

The longitudinal rib and the cross rib of the foot take a great deal of punishment during walking, particularly during the landing and push-off phases. The ligaments and the aponeurosis plantaris that directly support the two ribs are passive tissues that cannot be trained; instead, the muscles of the foot can and must be trained in order to reduce the risk of injury. Your feet do a great deal of work for you during walking, so give them some special attention each day and watch your strength improve over time.

Start with this simple exercise: Drop a towel on the floor, stand with one foot on the towel and one off, and try to pick up the towel with your toes. After several weeks, proceed to this next exercise, which will strengthen your foot muscles, toe joints, ankles and knees: Stand in a bucket filled with sand and squeeze the sand with your toes for 10 minutes.

Calf Raises (figure 18-a, 18-b)

Stand on the edge of a step with your heels hanging over so that your toes carry your weight. Slowly raise and lower yourself. Start with both feet and then try one foot at a time. You can add a light weight after a few weeks of single-leg raises. This drill improves the strength and flexibility of the lower leg muscle group.

Step-ups (figure 19-a, 19-b)

Find a sturdy bench you can step on that isn't too high (your knee shouldn't bend tighter than 90 degrees when your foot is on the bench). Step up onto the bench and stand up straight before you step down. Alternate your feet each time. This drill works the upper leg muscles and hip flexors.

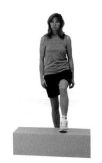

figure 19-a

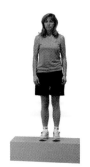

figure 19-b

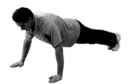

figure 20-a

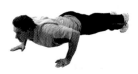

figure 20-b

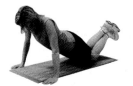

figure 20-c

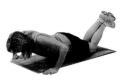

figure 20-d

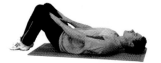

figure 21-a

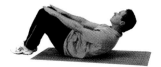

figure 21-b

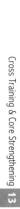

Upper and Mid-Body Strength Training

Achieving your personal goals may revolve around improving your core strength. Turn your attention to some core abdominal and pelvic strength.

Walkers get plenty of leg development through walking. Many walkers incorporate hill training or intervals for leg strength and some resistance weight training for the upper body. The muscles in your pelvis are continually stressed by walking. You need to spend some time on your abdominal and psoas muscles.*

*There are two psoas muscles on each side of the back. The larger of the two is called the psoas major and the smaller the psoas minor. The word "psoas" is Greek for loins, the muscles of the lower back.

The pelvis is the platform of your body. During walking it absorbs shock and transfers the weight of your torso and upper body to the legs. The stronger the platform, the better it absorbs the shock of each foot strike. Our body absorbs over three times our weight on each foot strike, so maintaining strong pelvic muscles will reduce the risk of injuries.

The abdominal muscles provide stability to the body, and the psoas create the impulse of energy that initiates leg movement. The abdominal muscles, the wash board muscles in our stomach area, are easy to identify and see. The psoas you cannot see. This long muscle works through the pelvis and inserts on the inside of the top of your thighbone. It is the primary initiator of your walking movement.

Push-ups (figure 20-a, 20-b, 20-c, 20-d)

Yes, your old phys-ed teacher was right: Push-ups are good for you. Push-ups work on all the upper body muscle groups, improving your walking form and posture. We all know how to do them; it's getting around to doing them that's a problem. This single exercise could replace a lot of time in the weight room if only we didn't find it so boring. Check off a daily 25 or so. Be sure to keep your back straight.

Sit-ups—the right way (figure 21-a, 21-b)

We have all seen the many infomercials on the benefits of the latest abdominal equipment on the market. Well, save yourself a few bucks; do this sit-up as part of your daily routine and those abs of steel will be yours! The great benefit of this sit-up is it works all the abdominal muscles from the rib cage through to the groin area. You too, could have that infomercial "six-pack belly."

Lie flat on your back with your knees bent and your feet flat on the floor. Be sure to do an abdominal tuck to flatten the small of your back against the floor. Now

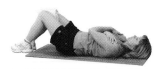

figure 22-a

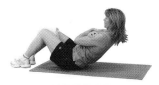

figure 22-b

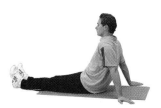

figure 23-a

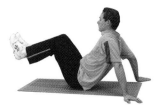

figure 23-b

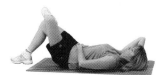

figure 24-a

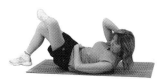

figure 24-b

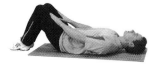

figure 25-a

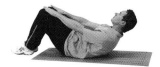

figure 25-b

extend your arms to put your hands on your thighs and then curl up your upper body, sliding your fingertips up to your knees. Keep the small of your back on the floor. Hold for a count of 10 and then lower yourself back to the floor. Start with about 25 repetitions and build from there.

The Crunch (figure 22-a, 22-b)

Place a towel between your knees and squeeze, contracting the inner thigh muscles. Curl your upper back towards your thigh muscles while doing a pelvic tilt; keep your lower back tight to the floor. Hold this position for 5–10 seconds. Return to the starting position, take a breath and relax, and then repeat a total of 10 times. This crunch will work the abdominals, the psoas and the adductor muscles of the inner thigh.

The Hipster (figure 23-a, 23-b)

Sit upright with your back perpendicular to the floor. Use your arms for support. Lean back and place your hands palms down on the floor, shoulder width apart. Keep your knees together, extend your legs straight out and then bring your knees back towards your chest. The heels are kept 6 inches off the ground throughout the routine. Repeat 20 times with a smooth and steady action. This builds strength in the psoas, hip flexors and lower abdominal.

The Crossed Leg Crunch (figure 24-a, 24-b)

Rest your right ankle on your left knee. Now curl your left shoulder up towards the inside of your right knee. Hold the crunch for 5–10 seconds, repeating 10 times. Now cross your legs the other way and repeat on the opposite side for 10 repetitions. This routine will strengthen your oblique stomach muscles and help prevent upper body rotation while walking.

Knee Slider (figure 25-a, 25-b)

Place the palms of your hands on your thighs. Slowly slide your hands towards your knees and lift your upper back. Contract your abdominals and keep your lower back tight on the floor. Curl and hold for a count of 5–10 and repeat 10 times. This strengthens your upper abdominals.

Do this circuit training three times per week and watch your walking times improve.

A Word about Weight Training

Balance the muscle groups. For most of our actions, muscles (or muscle groups) work in pairs, one moving the limb in one direction and the other moving the limb back to the starting position. This implies a certain balance between the muscle that does the action and the muscle that returns the limb to the starting position.

Most of us have a stronger and a weaker side. So when you are doing an exercise with both legs, one is working harder than the other. This imbalance tends to accentuate the difference in strength you started with. Isolating the leg by doing one leg at a time will balance off any strength variances in your legs.

Walkers and runners doing exercises for leg strength should make sure to avoid this strength difference. The cyclical nature of walking involves thousands of muscular contractions of each leg in each walk. Eliminating any significant strength difference between the two legs will help improve your performance.

Start doing leg exercises with both legs, to get comfortable with the action. After a few sessions reduce the weight and do the exercise with one leg at a time. You will quickly find which leg is stronger. Concentrate on the weak one; bring it up to the strength of the stronger one before you start working the strong leg again. Achieving balance in your leg muscles is a very worthwhile investment in our overall level of fitness.

Weight Training with Equipment
Why should I train this way?

The many benefits of resistance training include increased muscle strength, power, endurance and size. Additionally, resistance training can lead to increased bone density, reduced body fat, increased metabolic rate, lowered heart rate and blood pressure, improved balance and stability, enhanced performance of everyday tasks, and reduced risk of developing or improved management of medical conditions such as type II diabetes and arthritis.

American College of Sports Medicine (ACSM) guidelines for resistance training:

Frequency: two to three days per week

Intensity: choose 8–10 exercises that use the major muscle groups of the body

Duration: keep the movements slow and controlled for the most effective workout

Repetitions: one set of 8–12 repetitions (performing the movement 8–12 times consecutively)

Safety Tips
A major safety concern regarding resistance training is the use of proper body alignment and technique when completing an exercise. To ensure you are completing exercises properly and demonstrating proper technique, consult a personal trainer who can help you improve your form. When using free weights be sure to place collars on the ends of the bars to avoid weights sliding off.

For many free weight exercises it is essential to have a "spotter," so grab a buddy or ask a weight room attendant for assistance. They are there to help! Be sure to warm up your body before resistance training. Performing a few minutes of light cardiovascular exercise or performing the anticipated resistance exercise at a lighter weight will allow your body to prepare for the demands that are about to be placed on it.

Squat (figure 26-a, 26-b)
The squat is very effective in working the quadriceps, hamstrings and gluteal muscles. There are three main variations. Done properly, none of the variations is unsafe. For most walkers, the quarter squat is perfectly adequate for your needs. In a quarter squat the knees are bent to 90 degrees only.

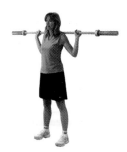

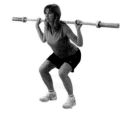

figure 26-a

figure 26-b

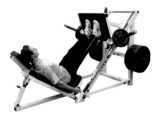

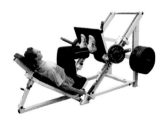

figure 27-a

figure 27-b

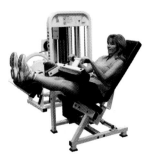

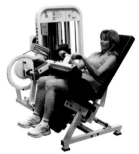

figure 28-a

figure 28-b

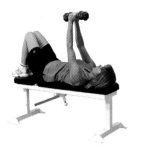

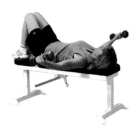

figure 29-a

figure 29-b

In a half squat, the knees are bent a little more so that the thighs are parallel to the ground. In a full squat, the knees are bent even more so that the buttocks are closer to the ground.

1. Use a squat rack designed to control the weight safely.

2. Stick your chest out and your shoulders back. This opens a "platform" on each shoulder where the bar can comfortably rest. In this position, the bar needs only to be steadied by your hands. Start with a comfortable position to begin the exercise. In this comfortable position, a pad or towel around the bar makes a difference for you. Do not load the bar onto the vertebrae in your neck.

3. The squat motion feels exactly like sitting down on a chair. Your feet are shoulder width apart. If you are at all unsure of your balance, put a chair underneath you so that you can literally sit down if necessary.

4. To be more stable, try putting each heel on a weight disk before you begin the exercise. Keep your weight on your heels.

5. Lower and raise the weight slowly. Maintain full control.

Leg Press (figure 27-a, 27-b)

Like the squat, the leg press is an exercise directly related to walking. You are pushing against a resistance with your feet, exactly like you do when you walk.

Leg press machines come in various forms. Generally, you sit and push pedals away from you with your legs, starting from a bent position until they are extended. Some even have you lying down and pushing the weight upwards, providing additional support for the back.

For walkers, a particularly effective form of the exercise is the reverse leg press. In the reverse leg press, you stand with your back to the pedals and support yourself by holding onto a pole behind the seat. You can then put a foot into one of the pedals and push the weight away from you in a motion similar to the push of a classic cross-country skiing action.

Leg Curl (figure 28-a, 28-b)

The traditional hamstring curl is done lying on your front on a bench. The feet fit under pads at the end of a bench allowing you to lift the weight by bending the knees. Some equipment allows you to sit upright, curling the legs underneath you. This has the advantage of isolating the hamstring muscle and removing the back muscles, which tend to creep into the exercise when you are lying down.

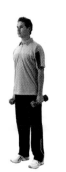

figure 30-a

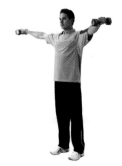

figure 30-b

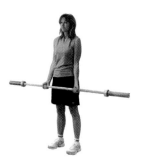

figure 31-a

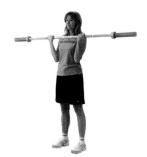

figure 31-b

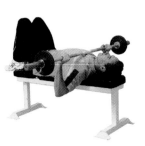

figure 32-a

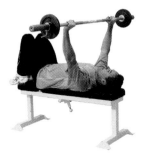

figure 32-b

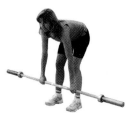

figure 33-a

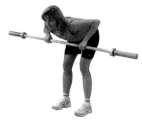

figure 33-b

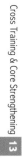

Dumbbell Fly (figure 29-a, 29-b)

Lie on your back on a bench with a dumbbell in each hand and your arms extended directly over your chest. Slowly lower the dumbbells directly out to the sides until your arms are parallel with the floor. Then bring your arms back slowly to the starting position, keeping your arms extended as you do.

Dumbbell Side-Raises (figure 30-a, 30-b)

Stand erect with your arms at your sides and a dumbbell in each hand. Raise the dumbbells upward from your sides, keeping your arms fully extended, until your hands are slightly above shoulder level.

Arm Curl (figure 31-a, 31-b)

Stand with your back straight, your head up and your feet slightly spread. Grasp the bar in an underhand grip (palms up) with arms fully extended. Then slowly curl the bar up to your chest. Hold for a count of two, and lower it to the starting position. Be careful to lower the bar slowly rather than let it drop from its own weight. Keep the bar under control at all times.

Bench Press (figure 32-a, 32-b)

Lie on your back on a bench or the floor with your back flat against the surface and the bar over your chest. Slowly press the bar straight up until your arms are fully extended, and then lower it slowly to the starting position.

Bent Row (figure 33-a, 33-b)

Bend over at the waist, keeping your back as flat as possible and your head up. Grasp the bar in a widely spaced overhand grip and raise it slowly to your chest. Lower it slowly to the floor and repeat. Bend your knees if necessary. Works the back.

Press Behind the Neck (figure 34-a, 34-b)

Stand erect with the bar resting on your shoulder. Press the bar directly up over your head and lower it slowly to the starting position. Works the posterior aspect of the shoulder.

Upright Row (figure 35-a, 35-b)

Stand with your back straight and your head up. Hold the bar in an overhand grip with arms fully extended. Keep your hands about 6 inches apart. Slowly raise the bar along the front of your body until your hands are under your chin. Lower it slowly to the starting position and repeat. Works the shoulder and neck.

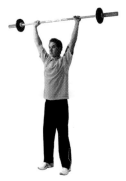

figure 34-a

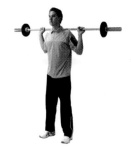

figure 34-b

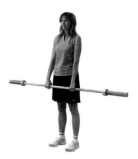

figure 35-a

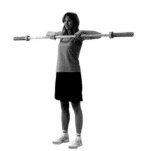

figure 35-b

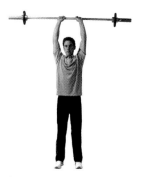

figure 36-a

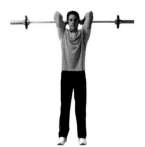

figure 36-b

Triceps Extension (figure 36-a, 36-b)

Stand erect with the bar pressed straight overhead. Your hands should be about 8 inches apart. Lower the bar slowly behind your head by bending your elbows. Slowly raise the bar to the starting position and repeat.

The weight exercises shown here train major muscle groups and, when used together, develop a good general muscle tone. If you are not sure how to do an exercise, ask a qualified professional or instructor for some help.

Nordic Walking Training

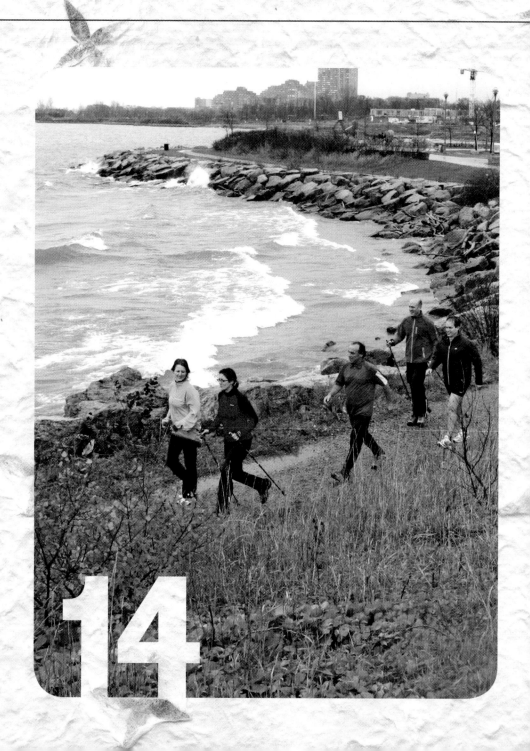

14

Nordic Walking Training

Nordic walking is an outdoor activity in which participants will utilize specially designed poles while walking on various types of terrain—asphalt, grass, dirt, gravel and sand. I would like to acknowledge Exel Sports and Mark Fenton, editor-at-large at *Walking* magazine, for providing the following information related to basic Nordic walking technique. They have had an active role in training the Walking Room staff on proper Nordic walking technique, and their contribution is appreciated.

Background

Nordic walking has a long history as a conditioning tool for competitive athletes. In the last decade, it has taken off as an ideal fitness activity for just about anyone. It is essentially walking with poles, using an alternating arm swing that is in opposition to the leg movement. Put more simply, Nordic walking looks like traditional (or classical) cross-country skiing without the skis and snow. This chapter summarizes how adding Nordic walking to your walking training routine can help with the four tenets of a successful program, listed here.

1. Effectiveness

A training program must assure that you attain the conditioning level necessary to reach your goal, whether a certain pace in a race or a specific level of fitness or weight loss. Nordic walking is a proven effective total body conditioner, used as off-season training by Nordic skiers for both aerobic and strength training.

2. Efficiency

Training should ideally provide the best possible conditioning in the least amount of time. This acknowledges that few of us are professional athletes, and most have obligations such as work, school and childcare. Why train three hours a day if 90 minutes will yield the same result? Nordic walking can be an efficient high-intensity workout, boosting energy expenditure over walking at the same speed by an average of 20% (as much as 45% if you pole vigorously, and even more during uphill intervals). And talk about efficient. Nordic walking combines aerobic and strength work into one session.

3. Safety

It's imperative to avoid injuries for a training program to be effective. Walking with poles can add stability on uneven ground or trails, poses no known elevated risk of injury to the upper body because the poles are so light, and can reduce the impact force on the lower extremity (as the poles bear some of your load.) This is especially true during downhill walking, which is when many hikers most appreciate using poles.

Health and fitness should never become a chore. That's why we set goals, train with others, participate in events, and, perhaps something we sometimes forget, should always be open to trying new things. New training loops, new walking partners, new races, and even new workouts can add a freshness that brings the fun back to your training. Nordic walking can be an especially fun alternative to mix into your routine because there is a technique involved. And it can be ideal to do on trails, fields or other more varied settings.

History and Benefits of Nordic Walking

For centuries humans have used walking sticks or staffs, and mountaineers have long used ski poles for rugged terrain and when carrying loads. In recent decades Nordic skiers have trained with their poles even when there's no snow on the ground to maintain upper body strength and overall fitness. In 1997 Exel, a ski pole manufacturer in Finland, worked with Suomen Latu, the National Federation of Popular Sports, to introduce Nordic walking to the Finnish population as an ideal fitness activity. The activity took off in Finland (it's estimated that over 15% of the population Nordic walk regularly and its popularity is growing rapidly across Europe. It has seen growth since 2000 in North America, and it is being introduced in New Zealand, Australia and other Pacific Rim nations.

Nordic Walking's Total-Body Benefits

Nordic walking on average increases the energy cost over walking at the same speed by about 20%. With vigorous poling, the increased energy expenditure can be 45% or more. The following muscles get a great workout during Nordic walking:

- back: upper and lower, especially the lats (latissimus dorsi), the wing muscles of the back, below the arms
- arms: especially the triceps (back of the upper arm) during the pushing movement
- shoulders: both front and back
- chest
- abdominals

The stride also tends to lengthen slightly with vigorous poling, increasing the workout for the quads (front of the thigh,) gluteal muscles and calves during the pushing phase of the stride.

Selecting and Strapping Into Nordic Walking Poles

Before using Nordic walking poles you need to select the correct size (they come in 5 cm increments) and know how to strap them properly onto your hands.

Selecting Your Pole Size

- While standing, with the pole upright on the ground and your hand on the grip, your elbow should be bent at a right angle. (Consult the sizing chart or visit www.nordicwalker.com for recommendations.)
- Select two sizes within the height range; err shorter for novice walkers.

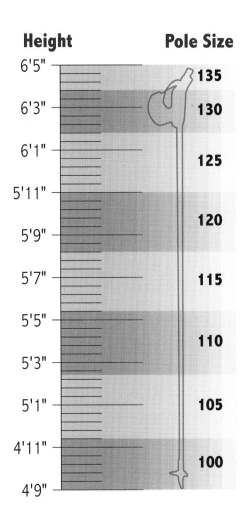

How to Strap in

* Unfasten the Velcro strap and let it hang open, untangled (poles are marked L & R).
* Insert your hand up through the strap from below until the strap surrounds the wrist. Grab the grip of the pole with your hand.
* Close the Velcro strap by wrapping it up over the wrist; as you attach it, you should see the "L" or "R."

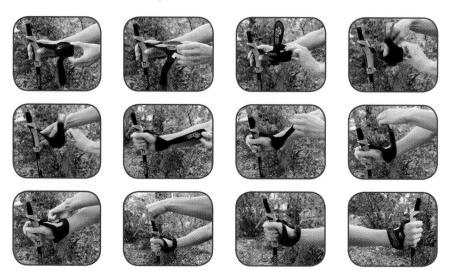

Correct Strap Adjustment

* While strapped into the pole, pull the webbing loop at the top of the grip upward; the plastic stopper will release from the grip.
* The webbing strap is now loose; pull it up so the strap snugly fits the hand. The goal is to have only a little slack between the grip of the pole and the hand.
* Re-insert the plastic stopper, pressing firmly into the hole atop the grip.

Nordic Walking Technique

Nordic walking is a natural walking movement, much like the classical or diagonal stride in cross-country skiing. Each arm swings forward with the opposite leg. So you plant a pole just about as the opposite heel strikes the ground (right pole with left foot, and vice versa) keeping the poles fairly close to your body and angled backward at about a 45-degree angle from your hand. As you drive back on the right foot, push back on the ground with the left pole, extending your arm backward and releasing the pole as you extend your ankle and push back on the ground with the ball of your foot and toes.

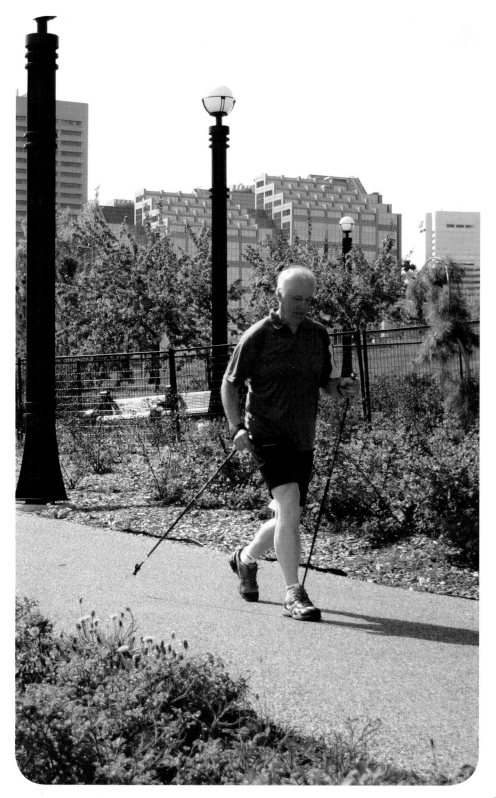

A simple way to learn Nordic walking is to use the Carry-Drag-Plant-Push progression. Begin on grass, dirt or gravel with rubber pole tips removed. The spiked pole tip will get better "grab," making the poling action more noticeable and push-off more effective.

Step 1: Carry (Before Strapping Into the Poles)

Grasp each pole at the middle of the shaft. Walk normally, with alternately swinging arms and legs. Feel the natural movement, get comfortable with weight of poles in your hands. Focus on long strides and full, even slightly exaggerated, arm swings.

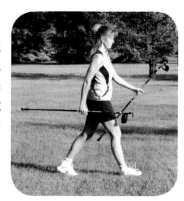

Step 2: Drag (Strap Into Your Poles)

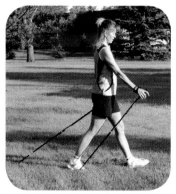

♦ While strapped in, release your hands so the poles hang at your sides by the straps.

♦ Walk normally, allowing your arms to swing freely forward and backward with a natural movement, opposite your legs; simply let the poles drag behind you.

♦ Increase or slightly exaggerate your arm swing, still not gripping the poles but letting them drag behind you. You'll feel the poles slightly grab or push on the ground as your arms begin their backward swing on each stride. Note that the poles are never upright but always angled backward.

Step 3: Plant

♦ Begin loosely grabbing the grips in each hand when your arms swing fully forward. You don't have to grab hard—just gently grasp the pole.

♦ Using the strap and grip, allow the pole to plant on the ground at about a 45-degree angle, pushing backward on the ground as you step forward with the opposite foot. Plant the pole tip roughly parallel to, and at about the same time as, the opposite foot.

- Don't put a death grip on the pole; release it as your arm swings back past your hips.

Step 4: Push

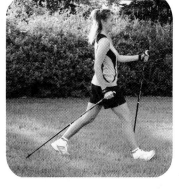

- Once the motion is comfortable, push backward on the poles more forcefully on each step—this will engage the triceps and latissimus dorsi muscles more completely.
- The overall goal is to rely more on the strap than the grip when pushing the pole backward into the ground, and to relax the hand and release the grip as the arm swings forward. This movement helps propel the body forward and lengthens the stride.

As you get more comfortable with the technique, extend your stride a little, add more forceful push-off (which will add a bounce to your step,) and maintain a slight forward body lean (just a couple of degrees) all the way from your ankles to your head. You'll feel your hips rotating a bit more, opposite the natural forward and back rotation of your shoulders, right hip and left shoulder forward at the same time, and vice versa. The result is that your torso—your stomach, chest, upper and lower back muscles—are really the engine that drives the movement, with both your legs and your arms (with poles) acting as the "wheels" that apply the force to the ground.

Building Nordic Walking Into Your Training Program

You can do as many different types of Nordic walking workouts as you can pure walking or running workouts. Nordic walking leads itself to long endurance efforts: up-tempo, fartlek and intervals, hill work and even plyometric (or power development) drills. Three specific workouts are offered here to build into your walking or running program. The idea is to create efficient workouts that help you meet your training goals in less time. Runners will also enjoy reduced injury risk by interspersing one or two days of low impact activity. Here are three specific workouts to sprinkle into your program. A typical approach is to insert them once or twice a week, alternating the workout types to complement your other running and walking workouts.

1. Endurance and General Strength

Easy to moderate pace, with normal Nordic walking movement. Begin with as little as 30 minute workouts, and build up to an hour or more.

14

2. Upper Body Strength and Improved Sub-Maximal Speed

Up-tempo (either moderate to vigorous pace or rolling terrain) with a more aggressive poling movement for 25 to 45 minutes. These workouts can help boost your anaerobic threshold.

Example workout: 2K easy warm-up; 25 minutes effort; 1K cooldown

3. Explosive Power and Speed

Very vigorous pace, hill repeats and/or explosive drills (such as bounding, skipping or running with a powerful poling movement) for 20–30 minutes, with the most powerful poling motion. A great workout to build anaerobic power for shorter races and to enhance pure speed.

Example workout: Warm up easily 2K; 6 x 200 m uphills with vigorous poling, easy, walks back down; 2K cooldown

Example workout: 2K warm-up; 8 x 50m drills, alternating jogging, skipping, running, bounding (easy 50 m recoveries); 1.5K warm down

As you create your own Nordic walking workouts to mix into your program, follow these rules:

+ As with running and walking, begin and end every workout with 5–10 minutes of easy Nordic walking to gradually warm up and cool down.
+ When adding bounding, skipping, or steep uphill intervals, start with just 25 to 50 meters of hard effort in the initial workouts; gradually build up to as much as 200 meters.
+ For more gradual uphills and running intervals, begin with 100 meters, building up to as much as 800 meters.
+ Plan a Nordic walk workout to take about the same amount of time as the running or walking workout that it replaces. So for walking workouts, the distance Nordic walked will be about the same or a bit farther (as you may Nordic walk faster than normal walking). When replacing a run with a Nordic walk, plan to reduce the distance by 30–45%, depending on your running speed.

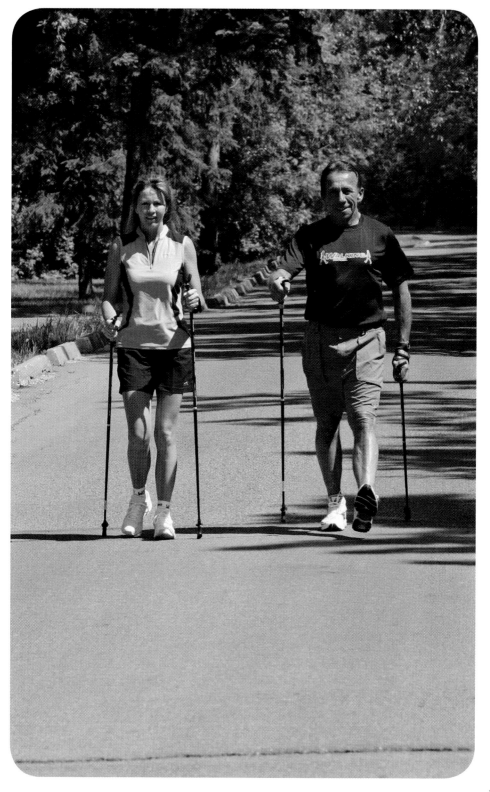

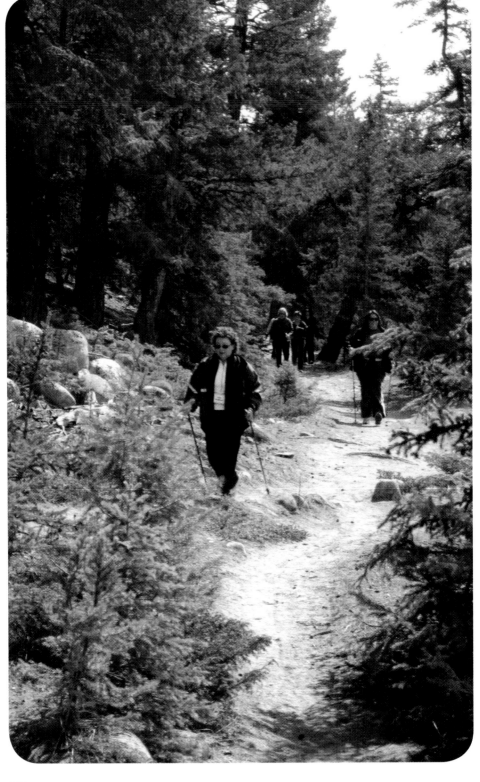

For 5K or 10K walk programs add one Nordic walk per week, alternating workout types 1 and 3. For example, weeks 3 and 4 of the 10K walking program:

10 km Walking Program Sample (recorded in km)

Week	Sun	Mon	Tue	Wed	Thu	Fri	Sat
3	6 Steady Walk	off	6 Nordic Walk Easy/Mod	off	6 Steady Walk	off	3 Steady Walk
4	8 Steady Walk	off	4 Nordic Walk w/Drills	3 Steady Walk	6 Steady Walk	off	3 Steady Walk

For half marathon or marathon walk programs, add three Nordic walks every two weeks, alternating all three workout types. For example, weeks 10 and 11 of the half marathon walking program:

Half Marathon Walking Program Sample (recorded in km)

Week	Sun	Mon	Tue	Wed	Thu	Fri	Sat
1	14 LSD Walk	off	5 Nordic Walk Easy/mod	12.5 Hills	off	6 Nordic Walk Up-tempo	5 Steady Walk
2	16 LSD Walk	off	5 Tempo	12 Nordic Walk w/Uphill Repeats	7 Steady Walk	off	5 Steady Walk

Nordic Walking Training

The Race in Race Walking

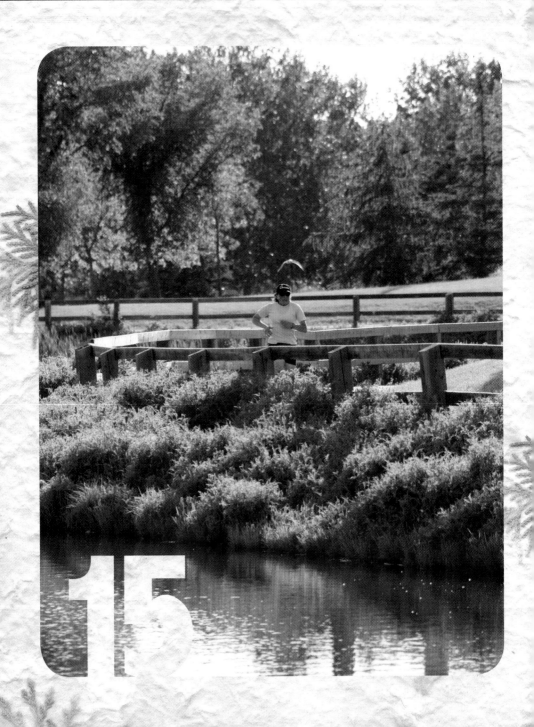

15

Understanding Race Walking

Specific race walk races differ greatly from the standard walking division in many of the running races and marathons. In running events with walking divisions, the walkers are asked to walk, not run, with the rules of doing so resting with those entered as a walker. Runners can walk, but walkers cannot run is the general rule. Implementation of this rule is generally done on the honor system. In most running events, there are no judges.

Specific race walk races can be held on a normal track or on a road course and are subjected to some very specific race walk rules and regulations. Road courses specifically for race walks often use a loop course for ease of judging and administration. Many performance races are required to use a loop. The loop length can be any distance up to 5000 meters, but 1000, 1250, 2000 and 2500 meters are the most common.

Distances for championship races are 20 km for men and women, and 50 km for men. Shorter distances, especially 5 km and 10 km, are common. Distances for younger athletes, and in indoor competition, can be as short as 800 meters and 1500 meters. Beginners are urged to use the shorter distances for their first ventures into competition. Even experienced athletes limit their racing at championship distances. Successful racing needs a quick rhythm, which is best developed in short races.

On the subject of race distance, if a course hasn't been measured by the Jones Counter method, it is not accurate. A Jones Counter measurement results in accuracy to 0.08% (8 m in a 10 km), and it's the only way a course can get certified under the present rules.

A race entry brochure will tell you a lot of the basic details. An entry fee is usually charged to help defray race expenses—generally these fees only pay a part of the total cost. Most often you will enter in advance.

Having entered, you show up on race day prior to race start time. Check the brochure carefully: sometimes you may have to pick up your race package before race day. Your race package may contain a whole range of information: forms for other races, technical information, your race number and timing chip. The number should be clearly identified as yours. At race package pickup check all your personal information for accuracy.

Your bib number is worn on the front and is clearly visible to all of the organizers and other athletes.

You warm up and come to the start line when called. In a race walk, you'll get instructions from the chief judge. You'll hear much of the same information at each race, but it's always worth paying attention just in case they add a particular point of information specific to this race.

You will notice a board facing you somewhere on the loop. This is the warning board, where the chief judge is stationed during the race. If warning notices come in from the judges recommending disqualification, the competitor's number will appear on the board with a mark beside it. On the third mark, the chief judge will approach the competitor with a red flag to remove him or her from the race. See the next section on the system of judging.

If this happens, you are supposed to leave the course and remove your number. All warnings are recorded; a good chief judge will consider it part of the job to talk to you. Figure out what your violation was because at least three people thought it had occurred. Work on it for the next race.

For most races, over about 5 km, there will be a water station, at least one per lap. If the race is less than 10 km, you may only get water. In races of 10 km and over, you can have personal supplements as long as you bring them yourself and put them on the refreshment table provided by the organizers.

It is against the rules to get refreshments other than from the official water station. In important races, this will be enforced, so it's a good idea to practice taking water.

Race results are generally posted shortly after the final walker crosses the finish line. It's considered good etiquette to stay for the awards presentation.

A thank you to the race director is genuinely appreciated after the race. But perhaps the greatest appreciation you can show is to give up one of your races per year and volunteer to work at the race. You'll be surprised at the variety of things there is to do and what you learn from the other side of the race, as a volunteer.

The System of Judging

Judging is carried out by a group of officials called race walk judges. For track races, there will normally be five, plus a chief judge. On the road, there may be up to eight plus a chief judge. In higher level races, the chief judge does not act as a working judge; he/she coordinates the work of all the other judges and administers the judging system. For other competitions, it is practical and normal for the chief judge to judge as well.

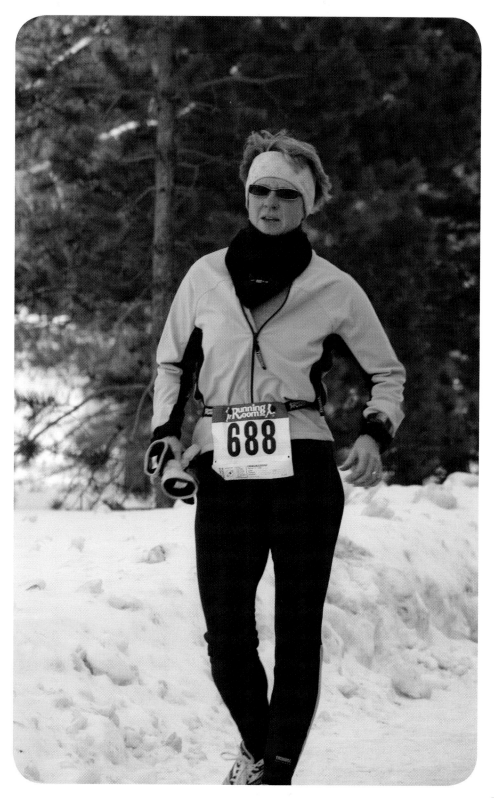

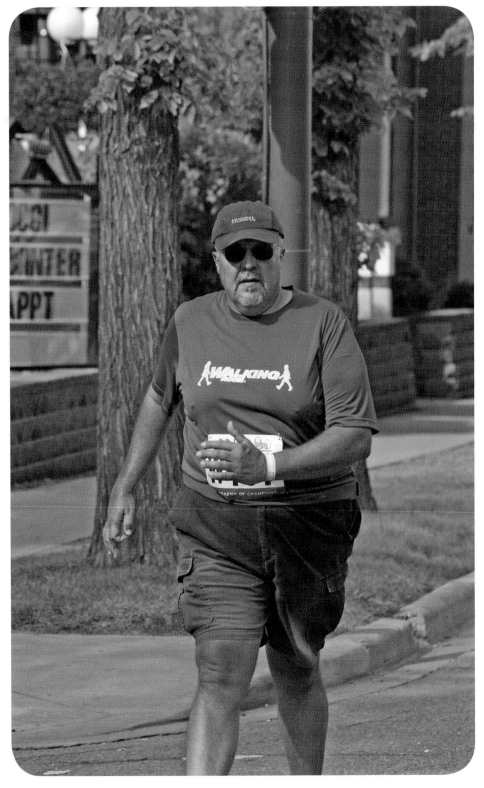

The System of Judging Is

1. It takes the opinion of three judges for an athlete to be disqualified.

   In international competition, the judges must come from three different countries.

2. Judges work independently: they do not consult with each other nor anyone else during a race. Judges transmit their recommendations to the chief judge.

3. Judging is done by the unaided human eye.

4. When a judge cautions an athlete by showing a white paddle, it simply may mean that the athlete is "in danger of infringing the rule." In other words, it may be "friendly advice" to the athlete: there is no required link with subsequent actions on the part of the judges.

   Experienced coaches teach athletes to use the judges' advice as constructive feedback.

5. If a judge feels that an athlete is definitely infringing the rules, especially to the extent that an unfair advantage is being gained over other competitors, the judge may decide that disqualification is warranted. The athlete is not informed until the chief judge has received a written proposal for disqualification from the judge. The chief judge then posts a mark against the athlete's number on a board visible to the athletes on each lap. This mark is called a "warning." In walkers' jargon, a warning is often called a "card" or a "red card."

6. If three warnings are received for the same athlete, the chief judge will remove the athlete from the race by showing a red flag. Disqualification may occur after the race is over.

7. The best judges consider their role is to ensure a competition that is fair for all. They do not feel that it is their role to evaluate technique against an "ideal" model.

Race walking in running races where the biggest group of walkers participate usually places the onus on the athlete to govern themselves—running races, thankfully, do not have formal judging system. Most walkers are in the race to walk their personal best times, with their own personal form, not under the subjective eye of a judge.

Selecting Your Training Program

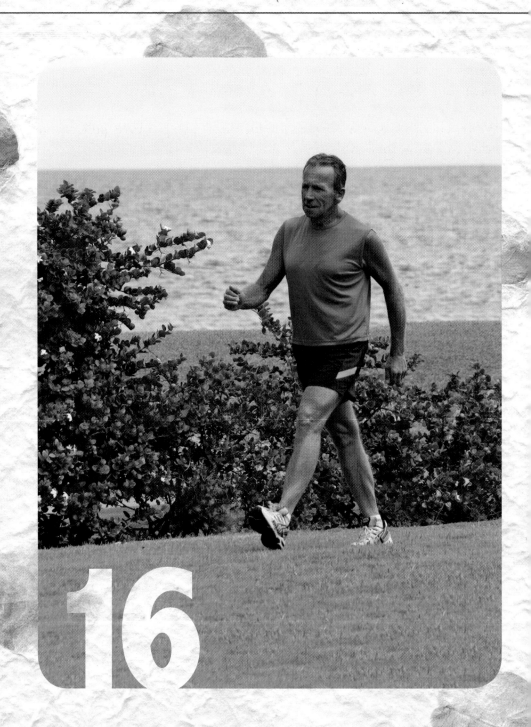

16

Selecting Your Training Program

Early in this book I pointed out the benefits of incorporating a walking routine as a part of your health and fitness planning. Setting up a program of consistently walking three to four days a week will immediately increase your energy level and stamina, relieve stress and tension, and help you sleep better. Over the long term a good walking routine will make you feel good about yourself and help you to achieve and maintain a healthy weight. When combined with healthy eating, walking will reduce the risk of developing heart disease, osteoporosis and certain cancers, and strengthen bones and muscles.

We are about to provide a number of different walking exercise programs to help you achieve these goals. First a word of advice that I feel is so important that it needs repeating:

See a Doctor First

Before starting any fitness program visit your doctor and tell them about your plans to start a walking program Your starting point is to assess your physical condition and then choose a program appropriate for your current level of fitness and one you find challenging, yet comfortable. Once you have begun the program, reassess your choice and if you feel you are overexerting, slow down. Alternatively, if you are not feeling some effect from your walking program, try one of the more advanced programs, walking at a faster pace and for longer distances.

Starting Point

In this chapter, we present programs for the beginner to advanced walker. We also offer a couple of maintenance programs for people with a strong walking base who are looking for a strong maintenance or fat-burning program. You will also see a number of programs put together for the athlete who may have a distance or time goal in mind. You will find programs focusing on 5 km, 10 km, half marathon and marathon distances. Don't be intimidated by these distances and programs. Many people need a distance goal to relate to rather than a time goal. As opposed to a goal of being able to walk for one hour, they are more motivated by a tangible distance, like being able to walk for 5 km. This book provides you with both options and you choose the one right for you.

Some walkers may already have a great base of walking and will use these programs to achieve such personal lifelong milestones as completing a marathon. Others may never be motivated to walk this distance and will focus on establishing a disciplined routine that is right for them. Whatever your fitness level or goals, there is a program for you. The walking programs presented in this chapter are grouped into three categories:

1. programs designed for people who are currently inactive

2. programs designed for people who are physically active on a regular basis

3. programs designed for people who have a fitness goal and may want to complete a certain distance and even compete in an event

The first group of sample programs is in the category of fitness walking. All these programs are time based: All workouts are based upon the number of minutes walked, as opposed to the total mileage. When starting, program participants have an easier time relating to the amount of time in an activity as opposed to the distance involved. Programs based strictly on time of activity are easy to work with and to schedule into your daily routine. Advancing in the program brings a more challenging distance goal, for example completing a 10K, half or full marathon, with higher daily mileage goals. By the time you are ready to take on these distance goals you will want to gauge your progress by total distance and pace per kilometer or pace per mile.

Training Program Workouts

Long Slow Distance

Long Slow Distance walks are the cornerstones of a distance-training program. Take a full minute to stroll for every 10 minutes of brisk walking.

These walks are done much slower than race pace (60–70% of maximum heart rate), so don't be overly concerned with your pace. The purpose of these walks is to increase the capillary network in your body and raise your anaerobic threshold. They also mentally prepare you for long races. Your body and mind adapt to walking for a long period of time.

A Note on LSD Pace

The pace for the long walk on the training schedule chart includes the stroll time. This program provides an upper end (slow pace) and bottom end (fast pace) to use as a guideline. The upper end pace is preferable because it keeps you injury free. Walking at the bottom end pace is a common mistake made by many walkers. They try to walk at the maximum pace, which is an open invitation to injury. From my career as a coach of runners and walkers I know of very few athletes who have been injured from walking too slowly, but loads of athletes who incurred injuries by walking or running too fast. In the early stages of the program it is very easy to walk the long walks too fast, but in the marathon or half marathon programs the long walks require discipline and patience. Practice your sense of pace by slowing down the long walks. Be specific in your training, walk fast on speed days and walk slow on distance days. Doing so you will recover faster and remain injury free.

Steady Walk/Stroll

The steady walk is a walk below targeted race pace (70% maximum heart rate). Walk at a comfortable speed; if in doubt, go slowly. The walk is broken down into components of brisk walking for 10 minutes and strolling for 1 minute. We encourage you to use the walk/stroll approach. Stroll breaks are a great way to stay consistent in your training. In addition to following the principle of training, stress and rest, the stroll breaks also divide your mental distance goal into a series of achievable goals.

Hills

Distance for the hill day is calculated as the approximate distance covered up and down the hill. Now, you will no doubt have to walk to the hill and back from the hill unless of course you drive to the hill. You will need to add your total warm-up and warm-down distance to the totals noted on the training schedule. I recommend a distance of 3 kilometers both ways to ensure adequate warm-up and recovery because hills put a lot of stress on the body. Hills are walked at tempo pace (80% maximum heart rate) and must include a heart rate recovery to 120 bpm at the bottom of each hill repeat.

VO2 Max

VO2 max is the volume of oxygen your body can obtain while training at your maximum heart rate. High VO2 levels indicate high fitness levels, allowing fit athletes to train more intensely than beginners. Interval training of tempo, fartlek and speed sessions improves the efficiency of your body to transfer oxygen-rich blood to your working muscles.

Tempo

Before starting tempo walks, include several weeks of once a week hill training to improve your strength, form and confidence. For the tempo walks, walk at 80% of your maximum heart rate for 60–80% of your planned race distance to improve your coordination and leg turnover rate. Include a warm-up and cooldown of about three to five minutes. These walks simulate race conditions and the effort required on race day.

Fartlek (Speed Play)

Fartlek walks are spontaneous walks over varying distances and intensity. Walk the short bursts at 70–80% of your maximum heart rate, if you are wearing a monitor. Conversation with others is possible, but you should notice increased breathing, heart rate and perspiration. Between these short bursts of hard effort, no longer than three minutes, add in recovery periods of easy walking to bring your heart rate down to 120 beats per minute. Speed play fires up your performance with a burst of speed. The added recovery/rest interval keeps the session attainable and fun.

Speed

Going back to our training analogy of "Building the House," speed training is nailing down the roof and one of the last things we do. You must have a sufficient base training and strength training period before tackling speed. Speed is simply fast walks over short distances, for example, five intervals of 400 meters, usually with a relatively long period of recovery to allow the unpleasant side effects of the anaerobic activity to diminish. In our training programs we factor in a 3 kilometer warm-up and 3 kilometer warm-down into the total distance to walk. I have seen many walkers come up injured when attempting speed work—inevitably as a result of walking too fast. In the training programs I have purposefully lowered the pace of your speed works to 95% of maximum heart rate. Higher rates generally cause deterioration in your form, and who wants to practice bad form. In these programs we use speed to fine tune, not to damage. It has proven very successful in all our programs.

Stroll Adjusted Race Pace

How do we arrive at a "stroll adjusted race pace"? When you are in the stroll portion of your walk/stroll repetition, you are moving slower than your average walk pace. When you are briskly walking, you are moving faster than your average walk pace. The stroll adjusted race pace factors in the variation in strolling and walking speed. The challenge is to know the average speed of your stroll pace. We have devised a formula to calculate moderate stroll pace, which allows us to determine the exact splits including walking and strolling pace. The effect of this calculation is that the stroll adjusted race pace is faster per kilometer than the average race pace. However, when combined with your slower stroll pace you will end up with your target race pace. You can go online at www.runningroom.com and print out your walk (stroll) adjusted pace bands for race day.

Fitness Walking Program

These 10-week sample programs are for beginner, intermediate and advanced walkers. Each program has two levels, allowing you to transition from one level to the next in a safe and consistent manner. The first level establishes a base level for number of walks per week, with the time of each walk and the recommended pace. The second level allows a smooth transition to increase the number of workouts per week, with time and pace increasing slightly.

Fitness Walking Programs

Maintenance Walking Programs

Training Schedule Guidelines

Selecting a Program

The schedules all contain a pace guide to help you select the program best suited to your current fitness level. The true beginner can start with a simple step count. At your normal walking pace, simply count how many steps you can walk comfortably in a minute. Count the steps for 10 seconds and multiply by six to get your step rate per minute. Match that step count to the guideline recommendation on the program. For example, if you have a step rate of 90–110 steps per minute you should start out in the beginner level 1 program. As your fitness improves you will see your step count improve as well. So if your steps per minute increase to 105–115 then you are ready for the beginner level 2 programs. If you have a pedometer and/or a Garmin GPS unit you will be able to determine your steps, speed and pace. Match those to the training program guidelines as an indicator of the program level you should be at.

Pace Guide

Training Level	Walk Speed Category	Step Rate (SPM)	Speed (kph)	Pace per km	Speed (mph)	Pace per Mile
Beginner	Active: Relaxed/Normal	90-110	3.22	18.38	2	30
		105-115	4.02	14.55	2.5	24
Intermediate	Power: Moderate	110-120	4.83	12.26	3	20
		120-130	5.67	10.34	3.5	17.1
Advanced	Athletic: Brisk	130-140	6.44	9.19	4	15
		140-150	7.41	8.06	4.5	13.2

The programs here give you plenty of options, so start with what you see as a target to achieve. If you are truly a novice walker and are looking for a starting point then start out in the beginner level 1 program. This program will help you establish a regular and safe walking routine with a slight weekly increase in your walking time. Your priority here is getting comfortable walking regularly during the week. Don't push the pace, as speed and time are not the goal. You are making a lifestyle change. Success comes from patience and consistency.

You can change levels at any time. You may decide just staying healthy is no longer the goal and that you want to improve your fitness. No problem. Try the intermediate walking programs or even the advanced programs, which will really challenge you with pace, duration and weekly walking days. You can also back up if the challenges of a program are too great and you start to fatigue. Move back to a program where you are comfortable with the pace.

No matter what program you are attempting we always incorporate pace breaks into the program. We call these pace breaks a stroll and encourage all walkers to take pace breaks. These periods of gentle walking are used as a recovery from the brisk walk efforts. You will find the one-minute pace breaks or stroll allow you to recover sufficiently to maintain a strong and consistent pace throughout the long distance walks.

Pay attention to rest days, they are just as important to your program's success, as the scheduled walking days. In *Chapter 3—Training Concepts & Terms*, I talk about progressive overload and describe how rest is critical to the body's ability to recover from workouts and to rebuild prior to the next period of high intensity. The programs are based upon the principle of stress and rest, and this formula will get you to your goal.

Walking Fitness: Beginners

This first program is for newly active walkers and is designed to establish a regular routine and start you off conservatively. The walking effort is a relaxed, normal pace, with lots of rest between workouts. Each week you will see improvement. You will slightly increase your walking times every two weeks.

Walking Fitness Beginner Level 1
Walking Effort Category: ACTIVE WALKING

Week	1	2	3	4	5	6	7	8	9	10
Minutes Walking	15	20	20	25	25	25	25	30	30	32
Walks per Week	3	3	3	3	3	3	3	3	3	3

Sample Program

Week	Sun	Mon	Tue	Wed	Thu	Fri	Sat	Weekly Total
1	15	off	off	15	off	15	off	45
2	20	off	off	20	off	20	off	60
3	20	off	off	20	off	20	off	60
4	25	off	off	25	off	25	off	75
5	25	off	off	25	off	25	off	75
6	25	off	off	25	off	25	off	75
7	25	off	off	25	off	25	off	75
8	30	off	off	30	off	30	off	90
9	30	off	off	30	off	30	off	90
10	32	off	off	32	off	32	off	96

Pace Schedule - Relaxed Pace

Step Rate (spm)	Speed (kph)	Pace Per km (min:sec)	Speed (mph)	Pace Per Mi (min:sec)
90–110	3.22	18:38	2	30:00

Note: Your actual speed and steps will vary depending on technique, terrain, and leg length.
Stroll: We encourage all walkers to take pace breaks—periods of gentle walking of any kind—as a recovery from the briskness of the periods of effort.

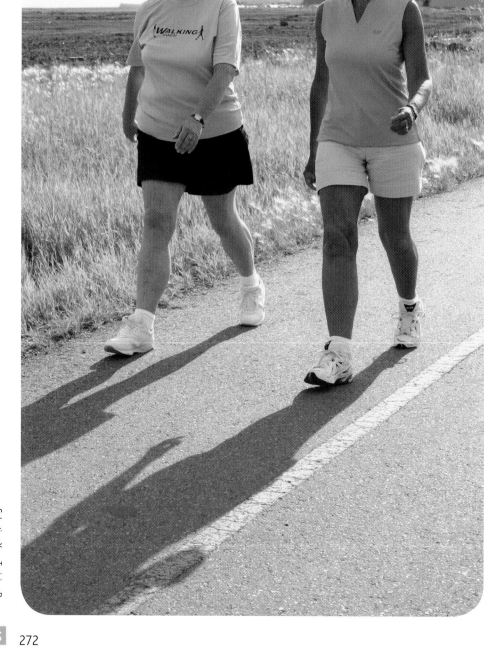

Walking Fitness Beginner Level 2 - Increased Effort*
Walking Effort Category: ACTIVE WALKING

Week	1	2	3	4	5	6	7	8	9	10
Minutes Walking	15	20	20	25	25	25	25	30	30	32
Walks per Week	3	3	3	4	4	4	4	4	4	4

Sample Program

Week	Sun	Mon	Tue	Wed	Thu	Fri	Sat	Weekly Total
1	15	off	off	15	15	off	off	45
2	20	off	off	20	20	off	off	60
3	20	off	off	20	20	off	off	60
4	25	25	off	25	25	off	off	100
5	25	25	off	25	25	off	off	100
6	25	25	off	25	25	off	off	100
7	25	25	off	25	25	off	off	100
8	30	30	off	30	30	off	off	120
9	30	30	off	30	30	off	off	120
10	32	32	off	32	32	off	off	128

Pace Schedule - Relaxed Pace

Step Rate (spm)	Speed (kph)	Pace Per km (min:sec)	Speed (mph)	Pace Per Mi (min:sec)
105–115	4.02	14:55	2.5	24:00

Note: Your actual speed and steps will vary depending on technique, terrain, and leg length.

* Covering similar distance but at a faster pace.

Stroll: We encourage all walkers to take pace breaks—periods of gentle walking of any kind—as a recovery from the briskness of the periods of effort.

16 Selecting Your Training Program

Walking Fitness: Intermediate

This second program starts to challenge you with an increase in days of the week committed to walking workouts and an increased faster pace. Each week you add time to your workouts, but pace and frequency remain fairly consistent.

Walking Fitness Intermediate Level 1
Walking Effort Category: POWER WALKING

Week	1	2	3	4	5	6	7	8	9	10
Minutes Walking	25	25	30	32	36	38	42	44	48	50
Walks per Week	3	3	4	4	4	4	4	5	5	5

Sample Program

Week	Sun	Mon	Tue	Wed	Thu	Fri	Sat	Weekly Total
1	25	off	off	25	25	off	off	75
2	25	off	off	25	25	off	off	75
3	30	30	off	30	30	off	off	120
4	32	32	off	32	32	off	off	128
5	36	36	off	36	36	off	off	144
6	38	38	off	38	38	off	off	152
7	42	42	off	42	42	off	off	168
8	44	44	off	44	44	off	44	220
9	48	48	off	48	48	off	48	240
10	50	50	off	50	50	off	50	250

Pace Schedule - Moderate Pace

Step Rate (spm)	Speed (kph)	Pace Per km (min:sec)	Speed (mph)	Pace Per Mi (min:sec)
110–120	4.83	12:26	3	20:00

Note: Your actual speed and steps will vary depending on technique, terrain, and leg length.
Stroll: We encourage all walkers to take pace breaks—periods of gentle walking of any kind—as a recovery from the briskness of the periods of effort.

Walking Fitness Intermediate Level 2 - Increased Effort*
Walking Effort Category: POWER WALKING

Week	1	2	3	4	5	6	7	8	9	10
Minutes Walking	25	25	30	32	36	38	42	44	48	50
Walks per Week	4	4	4	5	5	5	5	5	5	5

Sample Program

Week	Sun	Mon	Tue	Wed	Thu	Fri	Sat	Weekly Total
1	25	25	off	25	25	off	off	100
2	25	25	off	25	25	off	off	100
3	30	30	off	30	30	off	off	120
4	32	32	off	32	32	off	32	160
5	36	36	off	36	36	off	36	180
6	38	38	off	38	38	off	38	190
7	42	42	off	42	42	off	42	210
8	44	44	off	44	44	off	44	220
9	48	48	off	48	48	off	48	240
10	50	50	off	50	50	off	50	250

Pace Schedule - Moderate Pace

Step Rate (spm)	Speed (kph)	Pace Per km (min:sec)	Speed (mph)	Pace Per Mi (min:sec)
120–130	5.67	10:34	3.5	17:10

Note: Your actual speed and steps will vary depending on technique, terrain, and leg length.
*Covering similar distances but at a faster pace.
Stroll: We encourage all walkers to take pace breaks—periods of gentle walking of any kind—as a recovery from the briskness of the periods of effort.

Selecting Your Training Program

16

Walking Fitness: Advanced

The advanced programs build on the intermediate base. Advanced walkers work out at an even faster pace four to five times a week. The pace is brisk, so you need to be comfortable at the intermediate pace levels before moving to the advanced levels.

Walking Fitness Advanced Level 1
Walking Effort Category: ATHLETIC WALKING

Week	1	2	3	4	5	6	7	8	9	10
Minutes Walking	35	35	39	43	47	51	51	53	56	60
Walks per Week	4	4	4	4	4	4	4	5	5	5

Sample Program

Week	Sun	Mon	Tue	Wed	Thu	Fri	Sat	Weekly Total
1	35	35	off	35	35	off	off	140
2	35	35	off	35	35	off	off	140
3	39	39	off	39	39	off	off	156
4	43	43	off	43	43	off	off	172
5	47	47	off	47	47	off	off	188
6	51	51	off	51	51	off	off	204
7	51	51	off	51	51	off	51	255
8	53	53	off	53	53	off	53	265
9	56	56	off	56	56	off	56	280
10	60	60	off	60	60	off	60	300

Pace Schedule - Brisk Pace

Step Rate (spm)	Speed (kph)	Pace Per km (min:sec)	Speed (mph)	Pace Per Mi (min:sec)
130–140	6.44	9:19	4	15:00

Note: Your actual speed and steps will vary depending on technique, terrain, and leg length.
Stroll: We encourage all walkers to take pace breaks—periods of gentle walking of any kind—as a recovery from the briskness of the periods of effort.

Walking Fitness Advanced Level 2 - Increased Effort*
Walking Effort Category: ATHLETIC WALKING

Week	1	2	3	4	5	6	7	8	9	10
Minutes Walking	35	35	39	43	47	51	51	53	56	60
Walks per Week	4	4	4	5	5	5	5	5	5	5

Sample Program

Week	Sun	Mon	Tue	Wed	Thu	Fri	Sat	Weekly Total
1	35	35	off	35	35	off	off	140
2	35	35	off	35	35	off	off	140
3	39	39	off	39	39	off	off	156
4	43	43	off	43	43	off	43	215
5	47	47	off	47	47	off	47	235
6	51	51	off	51	51	off	51	255
7	51	51	off	51	51	off	51	255
8	53	53	off	53	53	off	53	265
9	56	56	off	56	56	off	56	280
10	60	60	off	60	60	off	60	300

Pace Schedule - Brisk Pace

Step Rate (spm)	Speed (kph)	Pace Per km (min:sec)	Speed (mph)	Pace Per Mi (min:sec)
140–150	7.41	8:06	4.5	13:20

Stroll: We encourage all walkers to take pace breaks—periods of gentle walking of any kind—as a recovery from the briskness of the periods of effort.

Note: Your actual speed and steps will vary depending on technique, terrain, and leg length.

*Covering similar distances but at a faster pace.

Walking a half hour a day or three to seven hours per week is associated with many health benefits. Once you have completed the fitness walking program you should be able to establish a daily routine of walking an hour a day, most days of the week.

Walk at least five days a week. We want to build a habit, so consistency is important. Spread out your rest days, such as making day 3 a rest day and day 6 a rest day. Each week, add five minutes a day to your walking routine.

If you find any week to be difficult, repeat that week rather than adding more time, until you are able to progress comfortably.

The Maintenance Walking Plan
Walking Effort Category: ACTIVE

Week	1	2	3	4	5	6	7	8	9	10
Minutes Walking	15	20	25	30	35	40	45	50	55	60
Walks per Week	5	5	5	5	5	5	5	5	5	5

Sample Program

Week	Sun	Mon	Tue	Wed	Thu	Fri	Sat	Weekly Total
1	15	15	off	15	15	off	15	75
2	20	20	off	20	20	off	20	100
3	25	25	off	25	25	off	25	125
4	30	30	off	30	30	off	30	150
5	35	35	off	35	35	off	35	175
6	40	40	off	40	40	off	40	200
7	45	45	off	45	45	off	45	225
8	50	50	off	50	50	off	50	250
9	55	55	off	55	55	off	55	275
10	60	60	off	60	60	off	60	300

Pace Schedule - Relaxed/Normal Pace

Your personal pace is entirely up to you, and you should, for the most part, be relaxed, steady and able to carry on a conversation. Stroll: We encourage all walkers to take pace breaks—periods of gentle walking of any kind—as a recovery from the briskness of the periods of effort.

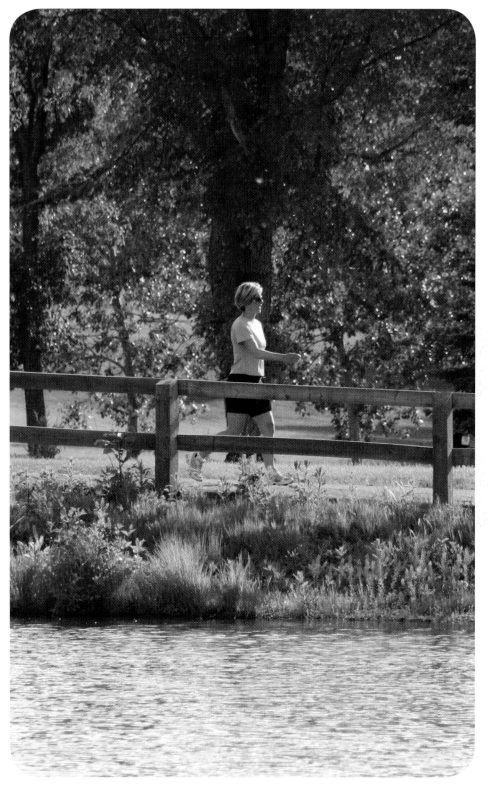

Maintenance Program: Lose Fat and Lose Weight

To lose weight and to keep it off, you need to get moving. This program is designed to burn calories and fat.

This workout gets the body to use stored fat for energy. At 60–70% of your maximum heart rate, 85% of your calories burned are fats. Walking slower burns a smaller percentage of fat. Walking at a moderate pace for 30–60 minutes burns stored fat and can build muscle to speed up your metabolism. Walking an hour a day is also associated with cutting your risk of heart disease, breast cancer, colon cancer, diabetes and stroke.

If your walking workout leaves you feeling sore or worn out the next day, take a day off. If this happens each day you walk, check your heart rate to be sure you are not overdoing it. Drop back up to 50% of the time walking each day and start building back up to the target goal by adding five minutes to each day's routing, each week.

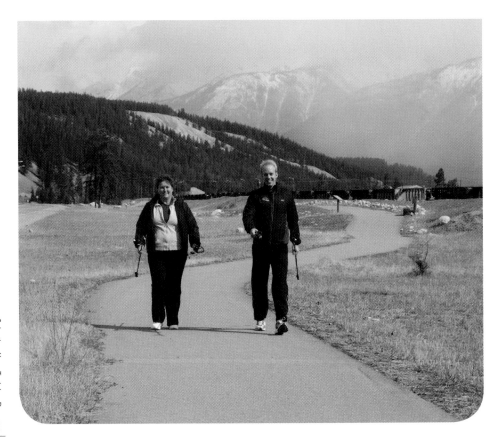

Maintenance Program: Lose Fat and Lose Weight
Walking Effort Category: ACTIVE

Week	1	2	3	4	5	6	7	8	9	10
Minutes Walking	30–60	30–60	30–60	30–60	30–60	30–60	30–60	30–60	30–60	30–60
Walks per Week	6	6	6	6	6	6	6	6	6	6

Sample Program

Week	Sun	Mon	Tue	Wed	Thu	Fri	Sat	Weekly Total
1	60	off	30	30	60	30	30	240
2	60	off	30	30	60	30	30	240
3	60	off	30	30	60	30	30	240
4	60	off	30	30	60	30	30	240
5	60	off	30	30	60	30	30	240
6	60	off	30	30	60	30	30	240
7	60	off	30	30	60	30	30	240
8	60	off	30	30	60	30	30	240
9	60	off	30	30	60	30	30	240
10	60	off	30	60	60	30	30	270

Pace Schedule - Relaxed/Normal Pace

Your personal pace is entirely up to you, and you should, for the most part, be relaxed, steady and able to carry on a conversation. Stroll: We encourage all walkers to take pace breaks—periods of gentle walking of any kind—as a recovery from the briskness of the periods of effort.

5 K Walking Programs

The 5 K programs start to move you from only time-based goals to distance goals as well. The athlete has a goal to be able to complete the total distance of 5 kilometers at a pace that feels comfortable to them.

Training Schedule Guidelines

Training Level	Step Rate (spm)	Speed (kph)	Pace per KM	Speed (mph)	Pace per Mile	Approximate time for 5k (min:sec)
Beginner	90-115	3.22-4.02	18.38-14.55	2-2.5	30-24	93.15–74.40
Intermediate	110-130	4.83-5.67	12.26-10.34	3-3.5	20-17.1	62.10–53.15
Advanced	130-150	6.44-7.41	9.19-8.06	4-4.5	15-13.2	46.35–41.25
Competitive	155-<	8.05-8.85	7.27-6.47	5-5.5	12-10.55	37.15–33.55

Selecting a Program

We have provided four programs for 5 K training: beginner, intermediate, advanced and competitive. We are still following the training program guideline from page 269 where the walking effort level ranges from a relaxed normal walking pace to a brisk pace. As you transition through the 5 K programs you will see that not only is the pace increasing but also the total time of each walk. Just as with the fitness walking programs, the 5 K programs allow you determine the schedule and pace best suited for you by choosing the pace schedule that best reflects where you are now. We have provide other benchmarks for you to use in determining which program is best suited to you—the approximate time needed to complete the distance of 5 kilometers.

5 K Training Programs

5 K Training: Beginners

This first program, for newly active walkers, is designed to establish a regular routine and start you off conservatively. The walking effort is a relaxed to normal pace with lots of rest between workouts. Each week you will see improvement. You will slightly increase your walking times every two weeks.

5 K Training - Beginner
Walking Effort Category: ACTIVE WALKING

Week	1	2	3	4	5	6	7	8	9	10
Minutes Walking	15	15	20	25	30	32	35	40	42	45
Walks per Week	3	3	4	4	4	5	5	6	6	6

Sample Program

Week	Sun	Mon	Tue	Wed	Thu	Fri	Sat	Weekly Total
1	15	off	off	15	15	off	off	45
2	18	off	off	18	18	off	off	54
3	20	20	off	20	20	off	off	80
4	25	25	off	25	25	off	off	100
5	30	30	off	30	30	off	off	120
6	32	32	off	32	32	off	32	160
7	35	35	off	35	35	off	35	175
8	40	40	off	40	40	40	40	240
9	42	42	off	42	42	42	42	252
10	45	45	off	45	45	45	45	270

Pace Schedule (min/km)

Step Rate (spm)	Speed (kph)	Pace Per km (min:sec)	Speed (mph)	Pace Per Mi (min:sec)	Approximate time for 5k (min:sec)
90–115	3.22–4.02	18:38–14:55	2–2.5	30–24	93:15–74:40

Stroll: We encourage all walkers to take pace breaks—periods of gentle walking of any kind—as a recovery from the briskness of the periods of effort.
Note: Your actual speed and steps will vary depending on technique, terrain and leg length.

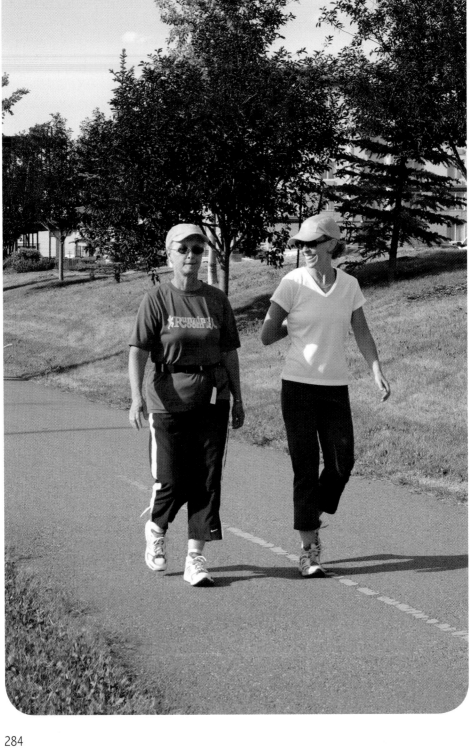

5 K Training: Intermediate

This second program starts to challenge you with an increase in days of the week committed to walking workouts, and those workouts are at a faster pace. Each week you add time to your workouts, but pace and frequency remain fairly consistent.

5 K Training - Intermediate
Walking Effort Category: POWER WALKING

Week	1	2	3	4	5	6	7	8	9	10
Minutes Walking	30	32	35	40	42	45	45	50	55	60
Walks per Week	3	3	4	4	4	5	5	6	6	6

Sample Program

Week	Sun	Mon	Tue	Wed	Thu	Fri	Sat	Weekly Total
1	30	off	off	30	30	off	off	90
2	32	off	off	32	32	off	off	96
3	35	35	off	35	35	off	off	140
4	40	40	off	40	40	off	off	160
5	42	42	off	42	42	off	off	168
6	45	45	off	45	45	off	45	225
7	45	45	off	45	45	off	45	225
8	50	50	off	50	50	50	50	300
9	55	55	off	55	55	55	55	330
10	60	60	off	60	60	60	60	360

Pace Schedule (min/km)

Step Rate (spm)	Speed (kph)	Pace Per km (min:sec)	Speed (mph)	Pace Per Mi (min:sec)	Approximate time for 5k (min:sec)
110–130	4.83–5.67	12:26–10:34	3–3.5	20–17.1	62:10–53:15

Stroll: We encourage all walkers to take pace breaks—periods of gentle walking of any kind—as a recovery from the briskness of the periods of effort.
Note: Your actual speed and steps will vary depending on technique, terrain and leg length.

Selecting Your Training Program

16

5 K Training: Advanced

The advanced programs build on the intermediate base. Advanced walkers work out at an even faster pace three to six times a week. The pace is brisk, so you need to be comfortable at the intermediate pace levels before moving to the advanced levels.

5 K Training - Advanced
Walking Effort Category: ATHLETIC WALKING

Week	1	2	3	4	5	6	7	8	9	10
Minutes Walking	45	47	50	55	57	60	65	70	75	60
Walks per Week	3	3	4	4	4	5	5	6	6	6

Sample Program

Week	Sun	Mon	Tue	Wed	Thu	Fri	Sat	Weekly Total
1	45	off	off	45	45	off	off	135
2	47	off	off	47	47	off	off	141
3	50	50	off	50	50	off	off	200
4	55	55	off	55	55	off	off	220
5	57	57	off	57	57	off	off	228
6	60	60	off	60	60	off	60	300
7	60	60	off	60	60	off	60	300
8	65	65	off	65	65	65	65	390
9	70	70	off	70	70	70	70	420
10	75	75	off	75	75	75	75	450

Pace Schedule (min/km)

Step Rate (spm)	Speed (kph)	Pace Per km (min:sec)	Speed (mph)	Pace Per Mi (min:sec)	Approximate time for 5k (min:sec)
130–150	6.44–7.41	9:19–8:06	4–4.5	15–13.2	46:35–41:25

Stroll: We encourage all walkers to take pace breaks—periods of gentle walking of any kind—as a recovery from the briskness of the periods of effort.
Note: Your actual speed and steps will vary depending on technique, terrain and leg length.

5 K Training: Competitive

The competitive 5 K schedule is much more difficult to maintain and not recommended for the inexperienced walker. The pace is very brisk, meaning the effort is difficult. Your step rate is very high and you will likely find breathing comfortably difficult if you are not properly prepared. You will definitely want to incorporate pace breaks within this schedule. Pace breaks are periods where you slow down the pace and stroll—a period of gentle walking to recover from the briskness of the higher level paces.

5 K Training - Competitive
Walking Effort Category: ATHLETIC WALKING

Week	1	2	3	4	5	6	7	8	9	10
Minutes Walking	60	62	65	70	72	75	75	80	85	90
Walks per Week	3	3	4	4	4	5	5	6	6	6

Sample Program

Week	Sun	Mon	Tue	Wed	Thu	Fri	Sat	Weekly Total
1	60	off	off	60	60	off	off	180
2	62	off	off	62	62	off	off	186
3	65	65	off	65	65	off	off	260
4	70	70	off	70	70	off	off	280
5	72	72	off	72	72	off	off	288
6	75	75	off	75	75	off	75	375
7	75	75	off	75	75	off	75	375
8	80	80	off	80	80	80	80	480
9	85	85	off	85	85	85	85	510
10	90	90	off	90	90	90	90	540

Pace Schedule (min/km)

Step Rate (spm)	Speed (kph)	Pace Per km (min:sec)	Speed (mph)	Pace Per Mi (min:sec)	Approximate time for 5k (min:sec)
155–>	8.05–8.85	7:27–6:47	5–5.5	12–10.55	37:15–33:55

Stroll: We encourage all walkers to take pace breaks—periods of gentle walking of any kind—as a recovery from the briskness of the periods of effort.

Note: Your actual speed and steps will vary depending on technique, terrain and leg length.

Selecting Your Training Program

16

10 K Walking Programs

Selecting a Program

Selecting the right 10 K program is important because you are now challenging yourself in the longer distances and committing more time and effort to your walking. In this section we will start out with a basic conditioning program based strictly on time as your primary measurement as opposed to distance. The goal of this program is to transition you into longer periods of walking in preparation for completing the 10 K distance. We will then move into the next set of programs and focus on distance and time goals. Your daily walks will be measured in distance achieved and suggest a very specific pace schedule for that distance. You will see that we offer five different time-goal training programs, each with increased effort and distance on your daily program. We do not recommend taking on the most challenging programs without first having a good training base. We recommend that you progress up the ladder from one schedule to the next to allow your body to adapt to the increased stress. If you start one program and do not experience it as challenging then certainly shift over to the next program.

The first program in the 10 K group of schedules is the 10-week 10 K conditioning program for beginners.

You will notice that the structured workouts in this stage of the program involve periods of effort over a comparatively short distance followed by a period of recovery. In *Chapter 4—Developing Your Walking Program* we go into detail about why we structure programs in this manner.

In the beginner 10 K conditioning program, we use a structure of interval training, which athletes often call "ins and outs." This is less precise than a traditional interval workout, where repetitions and recoveries are designed to be strictly measured and timed. With ins and outs, you don't stop during a set; you just slow down to a stroll and continue to your next starting point at a pace comfortable for you at the time. The repetition is generally quite short; you don't need to time it.

The ins and outs structure playful activity that is especially appropriate in the early stages of a walking program. This is because of the way in which we learn a new skill. Our brains need some time to get used to the new actions. In the initial stages of learning, we capture the skill for a few seconds and then seem to lose it.

This is quite normal. Our nervous system gets fatigued in a way physiologists still don't fully understand. However, we do know that a brief rest from a new skill allows us to try the skill again. We know that this pattern of brief rehearsal and recovery periods is more effective than continuing under fatigue. We also know that rehearsing a skill past the point of fatigue simply means that we are practicing the fatigued skill, not the desired one.

Once you are comfortable with the 10 K distance from the conditioning program you can move to the next set of programs, where we move away from only focusing on the time spent walking and begin to schedule based upon both distance and pace. We add in additional walk training types like hills, tempo and speed.

10 K Training Program (time based)

10 K Training Programs (recorded in km)

10 K Training Programs (recorded in mi)

10-Week 10 K Conditioning Program - Beginner

Week	1	2	3	4	5	6	7	8	9	10
Minutes Walking	30–44	30–44	40–54	40–51	40–66	30–70	50–80	50–80	50–90	40–44
Walks per Week	3	3	3	3	3	3	3	3	3	3

Week	Days per Week	Days of Week	Description	Walking Time	Session Time
1	Sunday Wednesday Friday	a	Warm-up: Stroll for 5 min. Walk for 25 min. Cool-down: Stroll for 5 min.	25	35
		b	Warm-up: Stroll for 10 min. 3 min. brisk walk followed by 2 min. Stroll; 2 min. brisk walk - 2 min. Stroll 1 min. brisk walk - 2 min. Stroll Repeat this combination 2 times. Cool-down: Stroll for 10 min.	44	
		c	Warm-up: Stroll for 5 min. Walk for 20 min. Cool-down: Stroll for 5 min.	20	30
2	Sunday Wednesday Friday	a	Warm-up: Stroll for 5 min. Walk for 20 min. Cool-down: Stroll for 5 min.	20	30
		b	Warm-up: Stroll for 10 min. 2 min. brisk walk followed by 2 min. Stroll; Repeat this combination 5 times. Cool-down: Stroll for 10 min.	40	
		c	Warm-up: Stroll for 5 min. Walk for 30 min. Cool-down: Stroll for 5 min.	30	40
3	Sunday Wednesday Friday	a	Warm-up: Stroll for 5 min. Walk for 30 min. Cool-down: Stroll for 5 min.	30	40
		b	Warm-up: Stroll for 15 min. 1 min. brisk walk followed by 2 min. Stroll; Repeat this combination 8 times. Cool-down: Stroll for 15 min.	54	
		c	Warm-up: Stroll for 5 min. Walk for 40 minutes Cool-down: Stroll for 5 min.	40	50
4	Sunday Wednesday Friday	a	Warm-up: Stroll for 5 min. Walk for 30 minutes. Cool-down: Stroll for 5 min.	30	40
		b	Warm-up: Stroll for 15 min. 5 min. brisk walk followed by 2 min. Stroll; Repeat this combination 3 times. Cool-down: Stroll for 15 min.	51	
		c	Warm-up: Stroll for 5 min. Walk for 40 minutes Cool-down: Stroll for 5 min.	40	50
5	Sunday Wednesday Friday	a	Warm-up: Stroll for 5 min. Walk for 30 minutes Cool-down: Stroll for 5 min.	30	40
		b	Warm-up: Stroll for 15 min. 3 min. brisk walk followed by 2 min. Stroll; 2 min. brisk walk followed by 2 min. Stroll; 1 min. brisk walk followed by 2 min. Stroll. Repeat this combination 3 times. Cool-down: Stroll for 15 min.	66	
		c	Warm-up: Stroll for 5 min. Walk for 50 minutes. Cool-down: Stroll for 5 min.	60	50
6	Sunday Wednesday Friday	a	Warm-up: Stroll for 5 min. Walk for 20 minutes. Cool-down: Stroll for 5 min.	20	30
		b	Warm-up: Stroll for 5 min. Walk for 60 minutes. Cool-down: Stroll for 5 min.	70	
		c	Warm-up: Stroll for 5 min. Walk for 30 minutes. Cool-down: Stroll for 5 min.	30	40
7	Sunday Wednesday Friday	a	Warm-up: Stroll for 5 min. Walk for 40 minutes. Cool-down: Stroll for 5 min.	40	50
		b	Warm-up: Stroll for 15 min. 5 min. brisk walk followed by 2 min. Stroll; 4 min. brisk walk - 2 min. Stroll 3 min. brisk walk - 2 min. Stroll 2 min. brisk walk - 2 min. Stroll 1 min. brisk walk - 2 min. Stroll Repeat this combination 2 times. Cool-down: Stroll for 15 min.	80	
		c	Warm-up: Stroll for 5 min. Walk for 60 minutes. Cool-down: Stroll for 5 min.	60	70
8	Sunday Wednesday Friday	a	Warm-up: Stroll for 5 min. Walk for 40 minutes. Cool-down: Stroll for 5 min.	40	50
		b	Warm-up: Stroll for 20 min. 2 min. brisk walk followed by 2 min. Stroll; Repeat this combination 10 times. Cool-down: Stroll for 20 min.	80	
		c	Warm-up: Stroll for 5 min. Walk for 70 minutes. Cool-down: Stroll for 5 min.	70	80
9	Sunday Wednesday Friday	a	Warm up: Stroll for 5 min. Walk for 40 minutes. Cool-down: Stroll for 5 min.	40	50
		b	Warm-up: Stroll for 5 min. Walk for 80 minutes. Cool-down: Stroll for 5 min.	80	90
		c	Warm-up: Stroll for 5 min. Walk for 65 minutes. Cool-down: Stroll for 5 min.	65	75
10	Sunday Wednesday Friday	a	Warm-up: Stroll for 5 min. Walk for 30 minutes. Cool-down: Stroll for 5 min.	30	40
		b	Warm-up: Stroll for 10 min. 3 min. brisk walk followed by 2 min. Stroll; 2 min. brisk walk - 2 min. Stroll 1 min. brisk walk - 2 min. Stroll Repeat this combination 2 times. Cool-down: Stroll for 10 min.	44	
		c	Event Day 10 K: Have fun and take care not to start out too quickly for yourself. Congratulations!		

Pace Schedule

Your personal pace is entirely up to you, and you should, for the most part, be relaxed, steady, and able to carry on a conversation.
Stroll: We encourage all walkers to take 'pace breaks' a period of gentle walking of any kind, used as a
recovery from the briskness of the periods of effort.

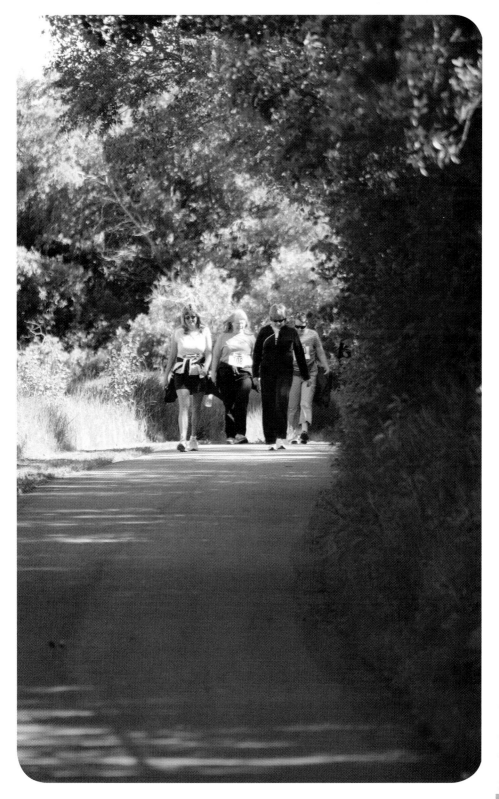

10 K Training Program Details

On the following pages you will find a variety of suggested training schedules. These schedules have been designed to help walkers to complete the event and/ or achieve specific time goals. The programs all follow the progressive structure as outlined in *Chapter 4—Developing Your Walking Program*. Long walks incorporate the 10 minutes of brisk walking and 1-minute stroll principle. In addition, you will see at the bottom of every training schedule a pace chart outlining the pace requirements for each walk. You can refer to *Chapter 2—Smart Walking* for a more detailed description of training methods. In addition *Chapter 3—Training Concepts & Terms* provides a nice review of the various workout requirements of a successful walking program.

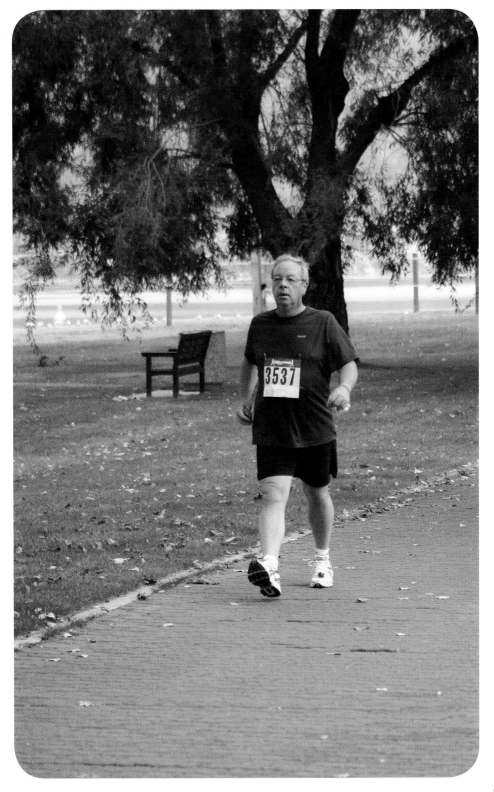

10 K Training - Beginner 2:00 (recorded in km)

Week	1	2	3	4	5	6	7	8	9	10
Distance Walking	10	15	18	19	17.5	18	20	22	23	17
Walks per Week	3	4	4	4	4	4	4	4	4	4

Sample Program

Week	Sun	Mon	Tue	Wed	Thu	Fri	Sat	Weekly Total
1	off	off	3 Walk/Stroll	4 Walk/Stroll	off	3 Walk/Stroll	off	10
2	5 LSD	off	3 Walk/Stroll	4 Walk/Stroll	off	3 Walk/Stroll	off	15
3	6 LSD	off	4 Walk/Stroll	4 Walk/Stroll	off	4 Walk/Stroll	off	18
4	7 LSD	off	4 Walk/Stroll	4 Walk/Stroll	off	4 Walk/Stroll	off	19
5	8 LSD	off	3 Walk/Stroll	2.5 3 x 400m Hills	off	4 Walk/Stroll	off	17.5
6	8 LSD	off	3 Walk/Stroll	3 4 x 400m Hills	off	4 Walk/Stroll	off	18
7	8 LSD	off	3 Walk/Stroll	4 5 x 400m Hills	off	5 Walk/Stroll	off	20
8	9 LSD	off	3 Walk/Stroll	5 6 x 400m Hills	off	5 Walk/Stroll	off	22
9	10 LSD	off	4 Walk/Stroll	5 Walk/Stroll	off	4 Walk/Stroll	off	23
10	6 LSD	off	3 Walk/Stroll	5 Walk/Stroll	off	3 Walk/Stroll	off	17
11	10 Race Day							10

Pace Schedule (min/km)

LSD	Steady Pace	Tempo/Hill/ Fartlek	Speed	Race Pace	Walk/Stroll Adjusted Race Pace
13:10–14:24	13:10	12:07	10:51	12:00	11:45

Pace: LSD & Walk/Stroll Interval = 10 min brisk walk, 1 min relaxed stroll

Hills: Hills are a distance of approximately 400 meters

Snags: If you find any week to be too difficult, repeat that week, rather than adding more time, until you are able to progress comfortably.

Pace Breaks: We encourage all walkers to take pace breaks—periods of gentle walking of any kind—as a recovery from the briskness of the periods of effort.

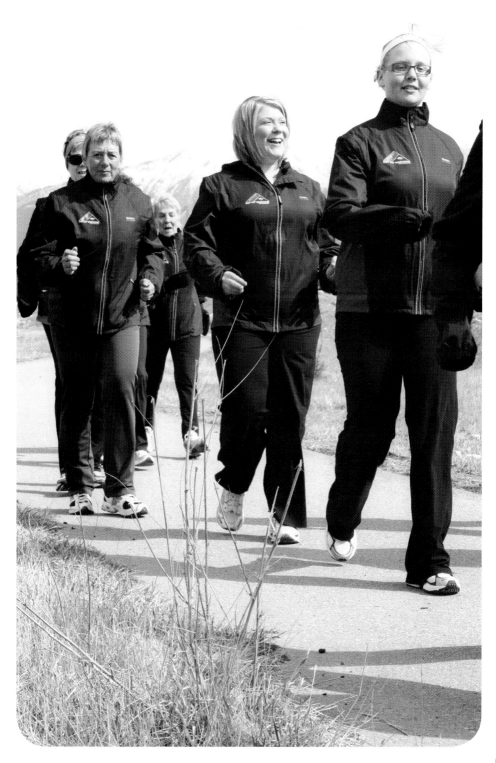

10 K Training - Beginner/Intermediate 1:50 (recorded in km)

Week	1	2	3	4	5	6	7	8	9	10
Distance Walking	14	21	21	26	27.5	30	33	35	38	29
Walks per Week	3	4	4	5	5	5	5	5	5	4

Sample Program

Week	Sun	Mon	Tue	Wed	Thu	Fri	Sat	Weekly Total
1	off	off	6 Steady Walk	off	5 Steady Walk	off	3 Steady Walk	14
2	6 LSD	off	6 Steady Walk	off	6 Steady Walk	off	3 Steady Walk	21
3	6 LSD	off	6 Steady Walk	off	6 Steady Walk	off	3 Steady Walk	21
4	8 LSD	off	6 Steady Walk	3 Steady Walk	6 Steady Walk	off	3 Steady Walk	26
5	8 LSD	off	6 Steady Walk	2.5 3 x 400m Hills	6 Steady Walk	5 Steady Walk	off	27.5
6	10 LSD	off	6 Steady Walk	3 4 x 400m Hills	5 Steady Walk	6 Steady Walk	off	30
7	10 LSD	off	8 Steady Walk	4 5 x 400m Hills	5 Steady Walk	off	6 Steady Walk	33
8	11 LSD	off	6 Steady Walk	5 6 x 400m Hills	8 Steady Walk	5 Steady Walk	off	35
9	11 LSD	off	8 Steady Walk	8 Tempo	5 Steady Walk	off	6 Steady Walk	38
10	13 LSD	off	8 Steady Walk	5 Tempo	off	3 Race Pace	off	29
11	10 Race Day							10

Pace Schedule (min/km)

LSD	Steady Pace	Tempo/Hill/ Fartlek	Speed	Race Pace	Stroll Adjusted Race Pace
12:14–13:27	12:14	11:14	10:00	11:00	11:00

Pace: LSD & Walk/Stroll Interval = 10 min brisk walk, 1 min relaxed stroll

Hills: Hills are a distance of approximately 400 meters

Snags: If you find any week to be too difficult, repeat that week rather than adding more time, until you are able to progress comfortably.

Pace Breaks: We encourage all walkers to take pace breaks—periods of gentle walking of any kind—as a recovery from the briskness of the periods of effort.

10 K Training - Intermediate 1:40 (recorded in km)

Week	1	2	3	4	5	6	7	8	9	10	11	12
Distance Walking	20	27	33	33.5	43	47	40	48	48	45.5	54	34
Walks per Week	4	5	5	5	5	5	5	5	5	5	5	5

Sample Program

Week	Sun	Mon	Tue	Wed	Thu	Fri	Sat	Weekly Total
1	off	off	6 Steady Walk	3 4 x 400m Hills	6 Steady Walk	5 Tempo	off	20
2	6 LSD	off	6 Steady Walk	4 5 x 400m Hills	6 Steady Walk	5 Tempo	off	27
3	10 LSD	off	6 Steady Walk	5 6 x 400m Hills	6 Steady Walk	6 Tempo	off	33
4	10 LSD	off	6 Steady Walk	5.5 7 x 400m Hills	6 Steady Walk	6 Tempo	off	33.5
5	13 LSD	off	8 Steady Walk	6 8 x 400m Hills	8 Steady Walk	8 Tempo	off	43
6	16 LSD	off	8 Steady Walk	7 9 x 400m Hills	8 Steady Walk	8 Tempo	off	47
7	13 LSD	off	8 Steady Walk	8 10 x 400m Hills	6 Steady Walk	6 Tempo	off	40
8	16 LSD	off	8 Steady Walk	8 4 x 400m Speed	8 Steady Walk	8 Tempo	off	48
9	16 LSD	off	8 Steady Walk	8 5 x 400m Speed	8 Steady Walk	8 Tempo	off	48
10	13 LSD	off	8 Steady Walk	8.5 6 x 400m Speed	8 Steady Walk	8 Tempo	off	45.5
11	16 LSD	off	8 Steady Walk	9 7 x 400m Speed	13 Steady Walk	8 Tempo	off	54
12	16 LSD	off	6 Race Pace	6 Race Pace	3 Steady Walk	off	3 Steady Walk	34
13	10 Race Day							10

Pace Schedule (min/km)

LSD	Steady Pace	Tempo/Hill/ Fartlek	Speed	Race Pace	Stroll Adjusted Race Pace
11:17–12:27	11:17	10:19	9:09	10:00	9:55

Pace: LSD & Walk/Stroll Interval = 10 min brisk walk, 1 min relaxed stroll
Hills: Hills are a distance of approximately 400 meters
Snags: If you find any week to be too difficult, repeat that week rather than adding more time, until you are able to progress comfortably.
Pace Breaks: We encourage all walkers to take pace breaks—periods of gentle walking of any kind—as a recovery from the briskness of the periods of effort.

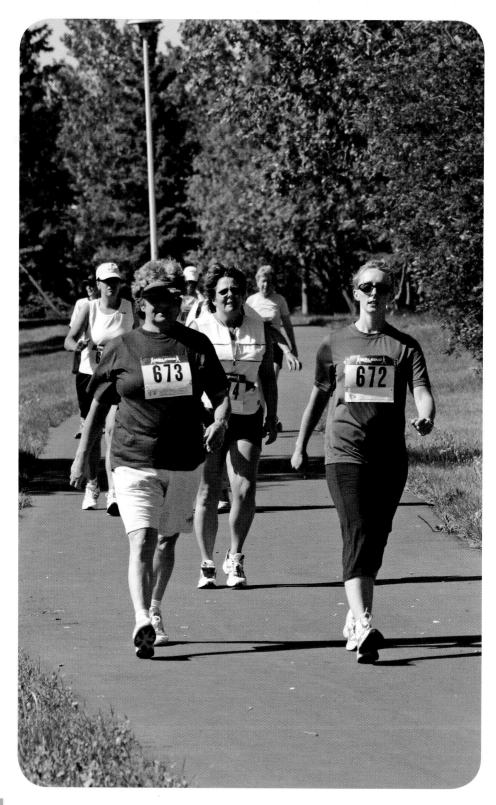

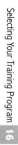

10 K Training - Intermediate 1:30 (recorded in km)

Week	1	2	3	4	5	6	7	8	9	10	11	12
Distance Walking	25	32	38	38.5	43	52	41	53	56	59.5	65	31
Walks per Week	5	6	6	6	5	6	5	6	6	6	6	5

Sample Program

Week	Sun	Mon	Tue	Wed	Thu	Fri	Sat	Weekly Total
1	off	off	6 Steady Walk	3 4 x 400m Hills	6 Steady Walk	5 Tempo	5 Steady Walk	25
2	6 LSD	off	6 Steady Walk	4 5 x 400m Hills	6 Steady Walk	5 Tempo	5 Steady Walk	32
3	10 LSD	off	6 Steady Walk	5 6 x 400m Hills	6 Steady Walk	6 Tempo	5 Steady Walk	38
4	10 LSD	off	6 Steady Walk	5.5 7 x 400m Hills	6 Steady Walk	6 Tempo	5 Steady Walk	38.5
5	13 LSD	off	8 Steady Walk	6 8 x 400m Hills	8 Steady Walk	8 Tempo	off	43
6	16 LSD	off	8 Steady Walk	7 9 x 400m Hills	8 Steady Walk	8 Tempo	5 Steady Walk	52
7	13 LSD	off	6 Steady Walk	8 10 x 400m Hills	8 Steady Walk	6 Tempo	off	41
8	16 LSD	off	8 Steady Walk	8 4 x 400m Speed	8 Steady Walk	8 Tempo	5 Steady Walk	53
9	19 LSD	off	8 Steady Walk	8 5 x 400m Speed	8 Steady Walk	8 Tempo	5 Steady Walk	56
10	22 LSD	off	8 Steady Walk	8.5 6 x 400m Speed	8 Steady Walk	8 Tempo	5 Steady Walk	59.5
11	26 LSD	off	8 Steady Walk	9 7 x 400m Speed	8 Steady Walk	8 Tempo	6 Steady Walk	65
12	13 LSD	off	6 Race Pace	6 Race Pace	3 Steady Walk	off	3 Steady Walk	31
13	10 Race Day							10

Pace Schedule (min/km)

LSD	Steady Pace	Tempo/Hill/ Fartlek	Speed	Race Pace	Stroll Adjusted Race Pace
10:18–11:25	10:18	9:24	8:18	9:00	8:51

Pace: LSD & Walk/Stroll Interval = 10 min brisk walk, 1 min relaxed stroll
Hills: Hills are a distance of approximately 400 meters
Snags: If you find any week to be too difficult, repeat that week rather than adding more time, until you are able to progress comfortably.
Pace Breaks: We encourage all walkers to take pace breaks—periods of gentle walking of any kind—as a recovery from the briskness of the periods of effort.

10 K Training - Advanced/Intermediate 1:20 (recorded in km)

Week	1	2	3	4	5	6	7	8	9	10	11	12
Distance Walking	25	36	38	41.5	46	52	47	53	56	57.5	65	31
Walks per Week	5	6	6	6	5	6	5	6	6	6	6	5

Sample Program

Week	Sun	Mon	Tue	Wed	Thu	Fri	Sat	Weekly Total
1	off	off	6 Steady Walk	3 4 x 400m Hills	5 Steady Walk	6 Tempo	5 Steady Walk	25
2	10 LSD	off	6 Steady Walk	4 5 x 400m Hills	5 Steady Walk	6 Tempo	5 Steady Walk	36
3	10 LSD	off	6 Steady Walk	5 6 x 400m Hills	6 Steady Walk	5 Tempo	6 Steady Walk	38
4	13 LSD	off	6 Steady Walk	5.5 7 x 400m Hills	5 Steady Walk	6 Tempo	6 Steady Walk	41.5
5	16 LSD	off	8 Steady Walk	6 8 x 400m Hills	8 Steady Walk	8 Tempo	off	46
6	16 LSD	off	8 Steady Walk	7 9 x 400m Hills	8 Steady Walk	8 Tempo	5 Steady Walk	52
7	19 LSD	off	8 Steady Walk	8 10 x 400m Hills	6 Steady Walk	6 Tempo	off	47
8	16 LSD	off	8 Steady Walk	8 4 x 400m Speed	8 Steady Walk	8 Tempo	5 Steady Walk	53
9	19 LSD	off	8 Steady Walk	8 5 x 400m Speed	8 Steady Walk	8 Tempo	5 Steady Walk	56
10	22 LSD	off	8 Steady Walk	8.5 6 x 400m Speed	6 Steady Walk	8 Tempo	5 Steady Walk	57.5
11	26 LSD	off	8 Steady Walk	9 7 x 400m Speed	8 Steady Walk	8 Tempo	6 Steady Walk	65
12	13 LSD	off	6 Steady Walk	6 Race Pace	3 Steady Walk	off	3 Steady Walk	31
13	10 Race Day							10

Pace Schedule (min/km)

LSD	Steady Pace	Tempo/Hill/ Fartlek	Speed	Race Pace	Stroll Adjusted Race Pace
9:18–10:21	9:18	8:27	7:26	8:00	7:48

Pace: LSD & Walk/Stroll Interval = 10 min brisk walk, 1 min relaxed stroll
Hills: Hills are a distance of approximately 400 meters
Snags: If you find any week to be too difficult, repeat that week rather than adding more time, until you are able to progress comfortably.
Pace Breaks: We encourage all walkers to take pace breaks—periods of gentle walking of any kind—as a recovery from the briskness of the periods of effort.

10 K Training - Advanced 1:15 (recorded in km)

Week	1	2	3	4	5	6	7	8	9	10	11	12
Distance Walking	34	45	56.5	52	68	77	79	72	68.5	75	59	37
Walks per Week	5	6	6	6	6	6	6	6	6	6	5	5

Sample Program

Week	Sun	Mon	Tue	Wed	Thu	Fri	Sat	Weekly Total
1	off	off	6 Steady Walk	4 5 x 400m Hills	8 Steady Walk	8 Tempo	8 Steady Walk	34
2	10 LSD	off	6 Steady Walk	5 6 x 400m Hills	8 Steady Walk	8 Tempo	8 Steady Walk	45
3	13 LSD	off	6 Steady Walk	5.5 7 x 400m Hills	13 Steady Walk	13 Tempo	6 Steady Walk	56.5
4	16 LSD	off	6 Steady Walk	6 8 x 400m Hills	8 Steady Walk	8 Tempo	8 Steady Walk	52
5	19 LSD	off	8 Steady Walk	7 9 x 400m Hills	13 Steady Walk	13 Tempo	8 Steady Walk	68
6	22 LSD	off	10 Steady Walk	8 10 x 400m Hills	16 Steady Walk	13 Tempo	8 Steady Walk	77
7	26 LSD	off	8 Steady Walk	8 4 x 400m Speed	16 Steady Walk	13 Tempo	8 Steady Walk	79
8	19 LSD	off	8 Steady Walk	8 5 x 400m Speed	16 Steady Walk	13 Tempo	8 Steady Walk	72
9	26 LSD	off	8 Steady Walk	8.5 6 x 400m Speed	16 Steady Walk	10 Tempo	off	68.5
10	26 LSD	off	8 Steady Walk	9 7 x 400m Speed	16 Steady Walk	8 Tempo	8 Steady Walk	75
11	26 LSD	off	8 Steady Walk	9 8 x 400m Speed	8 Steady Walk	8 Tempo	off	59
12	16 LSD	off	6 Race Pace	6 Race Pace	6 Steady Walk	off	3 Steady Walk	37
13	10 Race Day							10

Pace Schedule (min/km)

LSD	Steady Pace	Tempo/Hill/ Fartlek	Speed	Race Pace	Stroll Adjusted Race Pace
8:48–9:48	8:48	7:59	7:00	7:30	7:18

Pace: LSD & Walk/Stroll Interval = 10 min brisk walk, 1 min relaxed stroll
Hills: Hills are a distance of approximately 400 meters
Snags: If you find any week to be too difficult, repeat that week rather than adding more time, until you are able to progress comfortably.
Pace Breaks: We encourage all walkers to take pace breaks—periods of gentle walking of any kind—as a recovery from the briskness of the periods of effort.

Selecting Your Training Program

16

10 K Training - Beginner 2:00 (recorded in mi)

Week	1	2	3	4	5	6	7	8	9	10
Distance Walking	6.5	9.5	11.5	12	11	10	12.5	13.5	14	11
Walks per Week	3	4	4	4	4	4	4	4	4	4

Sample Program

Week	Sun	Mon	Tue	Wed	Thu	Fri	Sat	Weekly Total
1	off	off	2 Walk/Stroll	2.5 Walk/Stroll	off	2 Walk/Stroll	off	6.5
2	3 LSD	off	2 Walk/Stroll	2.5 Walk/Stroll	off	2 Walk/Stroll	off	9.5
3	4 LSD	off	2.5 Walk/Stroll	2.5 Walk/Stroll	off	2.5 Walk/Stroll	off	11.5
4	4.5 LSD	off	2.5 Walk/Stroll	2.5 Walk/Stroll	off	2.5 Walk/Stroll	off	12
5	5 LSD	off	2 Walk/Stroll	1.5 3 x 400m Hills	off	2.5 Walk/Stroll	off	11
6	3.5 LSD	off	2 Walk/Stroll	2 4 x 400m Hills	off	2.5 Walk/Stroll	off	10
7	5 LSD	off	2 Walk/Stroll	2.5 5 x 400m Hills	off	3 Walk/Stroll	off	12.5
8	5.5 LSD	off	2 Walk/Stroll	3 6 x 400m Hills	off	3 Walk/Stroll	off	13.5
9	6 LSD	off	2.5 Walk/Stroll	3 Walk/Stroll	off	2.5 Walk/Stroll	off	14
10	4 LSD	off	2 Walk/Stroll	3 Walk/Stroll	off	2 Walk/Stroll	off	11
11	10 Race Day							6

Pace Schedule (min/mi)

LSD	Steady Pace	Tempo/Hill/ Fartlek	Speed	Race Pace	Stroll Adjusted Race Pace
21:11–23:11	21:11	19:31	17:27	19:19	18:54

Pace: LSD & Walk/Stroll Interval = 10 min brisk walk, 1 min relaxed stroll
Hills: Hills are a distance of approximately 400 meters
Snags: If you find any week to be too difficult, repeat that week rather than adding more time, until you are able to progress comfortably.
Pace Breaks: We encourage all walkers to take pace breaks—periods of gentle walking of any kind—as a recovery from the briskness of the periods of effort.

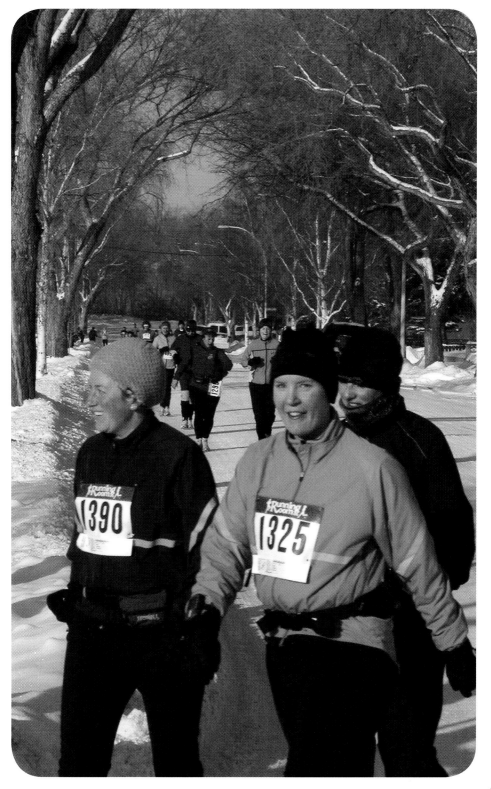

10 K Training - Beginner/Intermediate 1:50 (recorded in mi)

Week	1	2	3	4	5	6	7	8	9	10
Distance Walking	9	14	14	17	17.5	19	20.5	22	24	18
Walks per Week	3	4	4	5	5	5	5	5	5	4

Sample Program

Week	Sun	Mon	Tue	Wed	Thu	Fri	Sat	Weekly Total
1	off	off	4 Steady Walk	off	3 Steady Walk	off	2 Steady Walk	9
2	4 LSD	off	4 Steady Walk	off	4 Steady Walk	off	2 Steady Walk	14
3	4 LSD	off	4 Steady Walk	off	4 Steady Walk	off	2 Steady Walk	14
4	5 LSD	off	4 Steady Walk	2 Steady Walk	4 Steady Walk	off	2 Steady Walk	17
5	5 LSD	off	4 Steady Walk	1.5 3 x 400m Hills	4 Steady Walk	3 Steady Walk	off	17.5
6	6 LSD	off	4 Steady Walk	2 4 x 400m Hills	3 Steady Walk	4 Steady Walk	off	19
7	6 LSD	off	5 Steady Walk	2.5 5 x 400m Hills	3 Steady Walk	off	4 Steady Walk	20.5
8	7 LSD	off	4 Steady Walk	3 6 x 400m Hills	5 Steady Walk	3 Steady Walk	off	22
9	7 LSD	off	5 Steady Walk	5 Tempo	3 Steady Walk	off	4 Steady Walk	24
10	8 LSD	off	5 Steady Walk	3 Tempo	off	2 Race Pace	off	18
11	10 Race Day							6

Pace Schedule (min/mi)

LSD	Steady Pace	Tempo/Hill/ Fartlek	Speed	Race Pace	Stroll Adjusted Race Pace
19:41–21:38	19:41	18:04	16:06	17:42	17:17

Pace: LSD & Walk/Stroll Interval = 10 min brisk walk, 1 min relaxed stroll
Hills: Hills are a distance of approximately 400 meters
Snags: If you find any week to be too difficult, repeat that week rather than adding more time, until you are able to progress comfortably.
Pace Breaks: We encourage all walkers to take pace breaks—periods of gentle walking of any kind—as a recovery from the briskness of the periods of effort.

10 K Training - Intermediate 1:40 (recorded in mi)

Week	1	2	3	4	5	6	7	8	9	10	11	12
Distance Walking	13	17.5	21	21.5	27	29.5	25.5	30	30	31	30.5	22
Walks per Week	4	5	5	5	5	5	5	5	5	5	5	5

Sample Program

Week	Sun	Mon	Tue	Wed	Thu	Fri	Sat	Weekly Total
1	off	off	4 Steady Walk	2 4 x 400m Hills	4 Steady Walk	3 Tempo	off	13
2	4 LSD	off	4 Steady Walk	2.5 5 x 400m Hills	4 Steady Walk	3 Tempo	off	17.5
3	6 LSD	off	4 Steady Walk	3 6 x 400m Hills	4 Steady Walk	4 Tempo	off	21
4	6 LSD	off	4 Steady Walk	3.5 7 x 400m Hills	4 Steady Walk	4 Tempo	off	21.5
5	8 LSD	off	5 Steady Walk	4 8 x 400m Hills	5 Steady Walk	5 Tempo	off	27
6	10 LSD	off	5 Steady Walk	4.5 9 x 400m Hills	5 Steady Walk	5 Tempo	off	29.5
7	8 LSD	off	5 Steady Walk	4.5 10 x 400m Hills	4 Steady Walk	4 Tempo	off	25.5
8	10 LSD	off	5 Steady Walk	5 4 x 400m Speed	5 Steady Walk	5 Tempo	off	30
9	10 LSD	off	5 Steady Walk	5 5 x 400m Speed	5 Steady Walk	5 Tempo	off	30
10	8 LSD	off	5 Steady Walk	5 6 x 400m Speed	8 Steady Walk	5 Tempo	off	31
11	10 LSD	off	5 Steady Walk	5.5 7 x 400m Speed	5 Steady Walk	5 Tempo	off	30.5
12	10 Walk/Stroll	off	4 Race Pace	4 Race Pace	2 Steady Walk	off	2 Steady Walk	22
13	10 Race Day							6

Pace Schedule (min/mi)

LSD	Steady Pace	Tempo/Hill/Fartlek	Speed	Race Pace	Stroll Adjusted Race Pace
18:09–20:02	18:09	16:36	14:44	16:06	15:41

Pace: LSD & Walk/Stroll Interval = 10 min brisk walk, 1 min relaxed stroll
Hills: Hills are a distance of approximately 400 meters
Snags: If you find any week to be too difficult, repeat that week rather than adding more time, until you are able to progress comfortably.
Pace Breaks: We encourage all walkers to take pace breaks—periods of gentle walking of any kind—as a recovery from the briskness of the periods of effort.

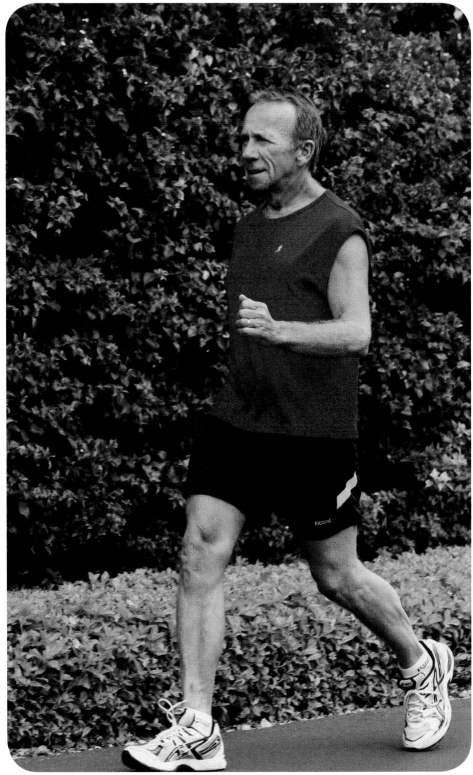

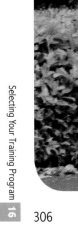

10 K Training - Intermediate 1:30 (recorded in mi)

Week	1	2	3	4	5	6	7	8	9	10	11	12
Distance Walking	16	20.5	24	24.5	27	32.5	26	33	35	37	40.5	20
Walks per Week	6	6	6	6	5	6	5	6	6	6	6	5

Sample Program

Week	Sun	Mon	Tue	Wed	Thu	Fri	Sat	Weekly Total
1	off	off	4 Steady Walk	2 4 x 400m Hills	4 Steady Walk	3 Tempo	3 Steady Walk	16
2	4 LSD	off	4 Steady Walk	2.5 5 x 400m Hills	4 Steady Walk	3 Tempo	3 Steady Walk	20.5
3	6 LSD	off	4 Steady Walk	3 6 x 400m Hills	4 Steady Walk	4 Tempo	3 Steady Walk	24
4	6 LSD	off	4 Steady Walk	3.5 7 x 400m Hills	4 Steady Walk	4 Tempo	3 Steady Walk	24.5
5	8 LSD	off	5 Steady Walk	4 8 x 400m Hills	5 Steady Walk	2 Tempo	off	27
6	10 LSD	off	5 Steady Walk	4.5 9 x 400m Hills	5 Steady Walk	2 Tempo	3 Steady Walk	32.5
7	8 LSD	off	4 Steady Walk	5 10 x 400m Hills	5 Steady Walk	4 Tempo	off	26
8	10 LSD	off	5 Steady Walk	5 4 x 400m Speed	5 Steady Walk	2 Tempo	3 Steady Walk	33
9	12 LSD	off	5 Steady Walk	5 5 x 400m Speed	5 Steady Walk	2 Tempo	3 Steady Walk	35
10	14 LSD	off	5 Steady Walk	5 6 x 400m Speed	5 Steady Walk	2 Tempo	3 Steady Walk	37
11	16 LSD	off	5 Steady Walk	5.5 7 x 400m Speed	5 Steady Walk	2 Tempo	4 Steady Walk	40.5
12	8 LSD	off	4 Race Pace	4 Race Pace	2 Steady Walk	off	2 Steady Walk	20
13	10 Race Day							6

Pace Schedule (min/mi)

LSD	Steady Pace	Tempo/Hill/Fartlek	Speed	Race Pace	Stroll Adjusted Race Pace
16:35–18:23	16:35	15:07	13:22	14:29	14:04

Pace: LSD & Walk/Stroll Interval = 10 min brisk walk, 1 min relaxed stroll
Hills: Hills are a distance of approximately 400 meters
Snags: If you find any week to be too difficult, repeat that week rather than adding more time, until you are able to progress comfortably.
Pace Breaks: We encourage all walkers to take pace breaks—periods of gentle walking of any kind—as a recovery from the briskness of the periods of effort.

10 K Training - Advanced/Intermediate 1:20 (recorded in mi)

Week	1	2	3	4	5	6	7	8	9	10	11	12
Distance Walking	16	22.5	24	26.5	29	32.5	30	33	35	36	40.5	20
Walks per Week	5	6	6	6	5	6	5	6	6	6	6	5

Sample Program

Week	Sun	Mon	Tue	Wed	Thu	Fri	Sat	Weekly Total
1	off	off	4 Steady Walk	2 4 x 400m Hills	3 Steady Walk	4 Tempo	3 Steady Walk	16
2	6 LSD	off	4 Steady Walk	2.5 5 x 400m Hills	3 Steady Walk	4 Tempo	3 Steady Walk	22.5
3	6 LSD	off	4 Steady Walk	3 6 x 400m Hills	4 Steady Walk	3 Tempo	4 Steady Walk	24
4	8 LSD	off	4 Steady Walk	3.5 7 x 400m Hills	3 Steady Walk	4 Tempo	4 Steady Walk	26.5
5	10 LSD	off	5 Steady Walk	4 8 x 400m Hills	5 Steady Walk	5 Tempo	off	29
6	10 LSD	off	5 Steady Walk	4.5 9 x 400m Hills	5 Steady Walk	5 Tempo	3 Steady Walk	32.5
7	12 LSD	off	5 Steady Walk	5 10 x 400m Hills	4 Steady Walk	4 Tempo	off	30
8	10 LSD	off	5 Steady Walk	5 4 x 400m Speed	5 Steady Walk	5 Tempo	3 Steady Walk	33
9	12 LSD	off	5 Steady Walk	5 5 x 400m Speed	5 Steady Walk	5 Tempo	3 Steady Walk	35
10	14 LSD	off	5 Steady Walk	5 6 x 400m Speed	4 Steady Walk	5 Tempo	3 Steady Walk	36
11	16 LSD	off	5 Steady Walk	5.5 7 x 400m Speed	5 Steady Walk	5 Tempo	4 Steady Walk	40.5
12	8 LSD	off	4 Steady Walk	4 Race Pace	2 Steady Walk	off	2 Steady Walk	20
13	10 Race Day							6

Pace Schedule (min/mi)

LSD	Steady Pace	Tempo/Hill/Fartlek	Speed	Race Pace	Stroll Adjusted Race Pace
14:58–16:40	14:58	13:36	11:59	12:52	12:27

Pace: LSD & Walk/Stroll Interval = 10 min brisk walk, 1 min relaxed stroll

Hills: Hills are a distance of approximately 400 meters

Snags: If you find any week to be too difficult, repeat that week rather than adding more time, until you are able to progress comfortably.

Pace Breaks: We encourage all walkers to take pace breaks—periods of gentle walking of any kind—as a recovery from the briskness of the periods of effort.

10 K Training - Advanced 1:15 (recorded in mi)

Week	1	2	3	4	5	6	7	8	9	10	11	12
Distance Walking	21.5	28	35.5	33	42.5	48	49	45	42	46.5	37	24
Walks per Week	5	6	6	6	6	6	6	6	5	6	5	5

Sample Program

Week	Sun	Mon	Tue	Wed	Thu	Fri	Sat	Weekly Total
1	off	off	4 Steady Walk	2.5 5 x 400m Hills	5 Steady Walk	5 Tempo	5 Steady Walk	21.5
2	6 LSD	off	4 Steady Walk	3 6 x 400m Hills	5 Steady Walk	5 Tempo	5 Steady Walk	28
3	8 LSD	off	4 Steady Walk	3.5 7 x 400m Hills	8 Steady Walk	8 Tempo	4 Steady Walk	35.5
4	10 LSD	off	4 Steady Walk	4 8 x 400m Hills	5 Steady Walk	5 Tempo	5 Steady Walk	33
5	12 LSD	off	5 Steady Walk	4.5 9 x 400m Hills	8 Steady Walk	8 Tempo	5 Steady Walk	42.5
6	14 LSD	off	6 Steady Walk	5 10 x 400m Hills	10 Steady Walk	8 Tempo	5 Steady Walk	48
7	16 LSD	off	5 Steady Walk	5 4 x 400m Speed	10 Steady Walk	8 Tempo	5 Steady Walk	49
8	12 LSD	off	5 Steady Walk	5 5 x 400m Speed	10 Steady Walk	8 Tempo	5 Steady Walk	45
9	16 LSD	off	5 Steady Walk	5 6 x 400m Speed	10 Steady Walk	6 Tempo	off	42
10	16 LSD	off	5 Steady Walk	5.5 7 x 400m Speed	10 Steady Walk	5 Tempo	5 Steady Walk	46.5
11	16 LSD	off	5 Steady Walk	6 8 x 400m Speed	5 Steady Walk	5 Tempo	off	37
12	10 LSD	off	4 Race Pace	4 Race Pace	4 Steady Walk	off	2 Steady Walk	24
13	10 Race Day							6

Pace Schedule (min/mi)

LSD	Steady Pace	Tempo/Hill/ Fartlek	Speed	Race Pace	Stroll Adjusted Race Pace
14:09–15:47	14:09	12:50	11:17	12:04	11:39

Pace: LSD & Walk/Stroll Interval = 10 min brisk walk, 1 min relaxed stroll
Hills: Hills are a distance of approximately 400 meters
Snags: If you find any week to be too difficult, repeat that week rather than adding more time, until you are able to progress comfortably.
Pace Breaks: We encourage all walkers to take pace breaks—periods of gentle walking of any kind—as a recovery from the briskness of the periods of effort.

Half Marathon Walking Programs

Half Marathon

"I'm only walking the half marathon," is a familiar quote I hear the day before many marathons across the country. Let's set the record straight: the half marathon is not half a race, and it is not called "only the half marathon." It is a challenging distance that gives most folks an equal sense of accomplishment as the full marathon. I like to call this event "the full" half marathon or better yet the 21.1K walk. Trust me, it is the full deal.

Occasionally, I like to tell walkers not to walk half marathons that are attached to full marathons for the very reason that the walkers often think they have only walked half a race. There are, however, many positive reasons to walk them: in most cases, the half marathon and the marathon start and finish at the same spot and for walking half the distance you get the same goodies at the finish, the same cheering finish-line crowd, the same T-shirt and the same good company to share your celebration.

Some folks really enjoy the half marathon distance; it challenges them but requires far less training and recovery than the marathon. Training for a half marathon requires going beyond normal fitness walking—it requires some additional time and commitment—but the celebration of the finish line is well worth the effort. The introduction into longer walks gets us back to the basics of long slow walking and the delights that come from doing them. We discover walking can be social, is great for burning fat and awakens us both mentally and physically.

Half Marathon Training Program Details

The training schedules on the following pages will help you prepare for a half marathon. Choose the schedule that best reflects your targeted finish time. There are two schedules for each time goal: the first one presents the training distances in kilometers; the second in miles. The half marathon is a serious distance; you must take your training seriously—so stick to the program. More is not necessarily better.

These schedules have been designed to help walkers complete the event and/or achieve specific time goals. The programs all follow the progressive structure as outlined in *Chapter 4—Developing Your Walking Program*. Long walks incorporate the 10 minutes walking/1 minute strolling principle that has made my programs so successful. In addition, you will see at the bottom of every training schedule a pace chart outlining the pace requirements for each walk.

You can refer to *Chapter 4—Developing Your Walking Program* for a more detailed description of training methods. In addition, *Chapter 3—Training Concepts & Terms* provides a nice review of the various workout requirements of a successful walking program.

Half Marathon Training - Beginner 3:15:00 (recorded in km)

Week	1	2	3	4	5	6	7	8	9	10	11	12	13	14	15	16	17
Distance Walking	9	20	21	21	23	24	24.5	26	30	34	38.5	40.5	37	42	42	44	25
Walks per Week	3	5	5	5	5	5	5	5	5	5	5	5	5	5	5	5	4

Sample Program

Week	Sun	Mon	Tue	Wed	Thu	Fri	Sat	Weekly Total
1	off	off	off	3 Tempo	3 Steady Walk	off	3 Steady Walk	9
2	7 LSD	off	4 Tempo	3 Tempo	3 Steady Walk	off	3 Steady Walk	20
3	7 LSD	off	4 Tempo	3 Tempo	4 Steady Walk	off	3 Steady Walk	21
4	7 LSD	off	3 Tempo	4 Tempo	3 Steady Walk	off	4 Steady Walk	21
5	9 LSD	off	4 Tempo	4 Tempo	3 Steady Walk	off	3 Steady Walk	23
6	9 LSD	off	5 Tempo	3 Tempo	4 Steady Walk	off	3 Steady Walk	24
7	10 LSD	off	4 Tempo	2.5 3 x 400m Hills	5 Steady Walk	off	3 Steady Walk	24.5
8	10 LSD	off	4 Tempo	3 4 x 400m Hills	5 Steady Walk	off	4 Steady Walk	26
9	12 LSD	off	4 Tempo	4 5 x 400m Hills	6 Steady Walk	off	4 Steady Walk	30
10	14 LSD	off	4 Tempo	5 6 x 400m Hills	6 Steady Walk	off	5 Steady Walk	34
11	16 LSD	off	5 Tempo	5.5 7 x 400m Hills	7 Steady Walk	off	5 Steady Walk	38.5
12	16 LSD	off	5 Tempo	6.5 8 x 400m Hills	7 Steady Walk	off	6 Steady Walk	40.5
13	12 LSD	off	5 Tempo	6 Fartlek	8 Steady Walk	off	6 Steady Walk	37
14	18 LSD	off	6 Tempo	4 Fartlek	8 Steady Walk	off	6 Steady Walk	42
15	18 LSD	off	6 Tempo	4 Fartlek	8 Steady Walk	off	6 Steady Walk	42
16	20 LSD	off	6 Tempo	4 Steady Walk	8 Steady Walk	off	6 Steady Walk	44
17	6 LSD	off	10 Steady Walk	6 Steady Walk	off	off	3 Steady Walk	25
18	21 Race Day							21

Pace Schedule (min/km)

LSD	Steady Pace	Tempo/Hill/Fartlek	Speed	Race Pace	Stroll Adjusted Race Pace
10:11–11:18	10:11	9:17	8:12	9:15	9:07

Pace: LSD & Walk/Stroll Interval = 10 min brisk walk, 1 min relaxed stroll

Hills: Hills are a distance of approximately 400 meters

Snags: If you find any week to be too difficult, repeat that week rather than adding more time, until you are able to progress comfortably.

Pace Breaks: We encourage all walkers to take pace breaks—periods of gentle walking of any kind—as a recovery from the briskness of the periods of effort.

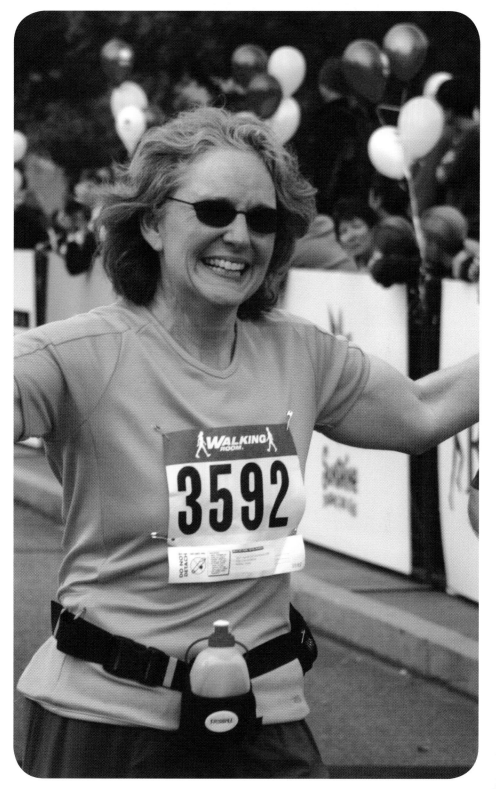

16 Selecting Your Training Program

Half Marathon Training - Intermediate 3:00:00 (recorded in km)

Week	1	2	3	4	5	6	7	8	9	10	11	12	13	14	15	16	17
Distance Walking	9	20	21	21	23	23	24.5	26	30	34	38.5	40.5	37	42	42	44	25
Walks per Week	3	5	5	5	5	5	5	5	5	5	5	5	5	5	5	5	4

Sample Program

Week	Sun	Mon	Tue	Wed	Thu	Fri	Sat	Weekly Total
1	off	off	off	3 Tempo	3 Steady Walk	off	3 Steady Walk	9
2	7 LSD	off	4 Tempo	3 Tempo	3 Steady Walk	off	3 Steady Walk	20
3	7 LSD	off	4 Tempo	3 Tempo	4 Steady Walk	off	3 Steady Walk	21
4	7 LSD	off	3 Tempo	4 Tempo	3 Steady Walk	off	4 Steady Walk	21
5	9 LSD	off	4 Tempo	4 Tempo	3 Steady Walk	off	3 Steady Walk	23
6	9 LSD	off	5 Tempo	3 Tempo	3 Steady Walk	off	3 Steady Walk	23
7	10 LSD	off	4 Tempo	2.5 3 x 400m Hills	5 Steady Walk	off	3 Steady Walk	24.5
8	10 LSD	off	4 Tempo	3 4 x 400m Hills	5 Steady Walk	off	4 Steady Walk	26
9	12 LSD	off	4 Tempo	4 5 x 400m Hills	6 Steady Walk	off	4 Steady Walk	30
10	14 LSD	off	4 Tempo	5 6 x 400m Hills	6 Steady Walk	off	5 Steady Walk	34
11	16 LSD	off	5 Tempo	5.5 7 x 400m Hills	7 Steady Walk	off	5 Steady Walk	38.5
12	16 LSD	off	5 Tempo	6.5 8 x 400m Hills	7 Steady Walk	off	6 Steady Walk	40.5
13	12 LSD	off	5 Tempo	6 Fartlek	8 Steady Walk	off	6 Steady Walk	37
14	18 LSD	off	6 Tempo	4 Fartlek	8 Steady Walk	off	6 Steady Walk	42
15	18 LSD	off	6 Tempo	4 Fartlek	8 Steady Walk	off	6 Steady Walk	42
16	20 LSD	off	6 Tempo	4 Steady Walk	8 Steady Walk	off	6 Steady Walk	44
17	6 LSD	off	10 Steady Walk	6 Active Walking	off	off	3 Steady Walk	25
18	21 Race Day							21

Pace Schedule (min/km)

LSD	Steady Pace	Tempo/Hill/Fartlek	Speed	Race Pace	Stroll Adjusted Race Pace
9:29–10:33	9:29	8:37	7:36	8:32	8:21

Pace: LSD & Walk/Stroll Interval = 10 min brisk walk, 1 min relaxed stroll

Hills: Hills are a distance of approximately 400 meters

Snags: If you find any week to be too difficult, repeat that week rather than adding more time, until you are able to progress comfortably.

Pace Breaks: We encourage all walkers to take pace breaks—periods of gentle walking of any kind—as a recovery from the briskness of the periods of effort.

Half Marathon Training - Advanced 2:45:00 (recorded in km)

Week	1	2	3	4	5	6	7	8	9	10	11	12	13	14	15	16	17
Distance Walking	9	20	21	21	23	24	24.5	26	30	34	38.5	40	38	44	42	46	25
Walks per Week	3	5	5	5	5	5	5	5	5	5	5	5	5	5	5	5	4

Sample Program

Week	Sun	Mon	Tue	Wed	Thu	Fri	Sat	Weekly Total
1	off	off	off	3 Tempo	3 Steady Walk	off	3 Steady Walk	9
2	7 LSD	off	4 Tempo	3 Tempo	3 Steady Walk	off	3 Steady Walk	20
3	7 LSD	off	4 Tempo	3 Tempo	3 Steady Walk	off	3 Steady Walk	21
4	7 LSD	off	3 Tempo	4 Tempo	3 Steady Walk	off	4 Steady Walk	21
5	9 LSD	off	4 Tempo	4 Tempo	3 Steady Walk	off	3 Steady Walk	23
6	9 LSD	off	5 Tempo	3 Tempo	4 Steady Walk	off	3 Steady Walk	24
7	10 LSD	off	4 Tempo	2.5 3 x 400m Hills	5 Steady Walk	off	3 Steady Walk	24.5
8	10 LSD	off	4 Tempo	3 4 x 400m Hills	5 Steady Walk	off	4 Steady Walk	26
9	12 LSD	off	4 Tempo	4 5 x 400m Hills	6 Steady Walk	off	4 Steady Walk	30
10	14 LSD	off	4 Tempo	5 6 x 400m Hills	6 Steady Walk	off	5 Steady Walk	34
11	16 LSD	off	5 Tempo	5.5 7 x 400m Hills	7 Steady Walk	off	5 Steady Walk	38.5
12	16 LSD	off	5 Tempo	6 8 x 400m Hills	7 Steady Walk	off	6 Steady Walk	40
13	12 LSD	off	5 Tempo	7 9 x 400m Hills	8 Steady Walk	off	6 Steady Walk	38
14	18 LSD	off	6 Tempo	4 Fartlek	8 Steady Walk	off	6 Steady Walk	42
15	18 LSD	off	6 Tempo	4 Fartlek	8 Steady Walk	off	6 Steady Walk	42
16	20 LSD	off	6 Tempo	4 Fartlek	8 Steady Walk	off	6 Race Pace	44
17	6 LSD	off	10 Steady Walk	6 Active Walk	off	off	3 Steady Walk	25
18	21 Race Day							21

Pace Schedule (min/km)

LSD	Steady Pace	Tempo/Hill/Fartlek	Speed	Race Pace	Stroll Adjusted Race Pace
8:46–9:47	8:46	7:57	6:59	7:49	7:36

Pace: LSD & Walk/Stroll Interval = 10 min brisk walk, 1 min relaxed stroll
Hills: Hills are a distance of approximately 400 meters
Snags: If you find any week to be too difficult, repeat that week rather than adding more time, until you are able to progress comfortably.
Pace Breaks: We encourage all walkers to take pace breaks—periods of gentle walking of any kind—as a recovery from the briskness of the periods of effort.

16 Selecting Your Training Program

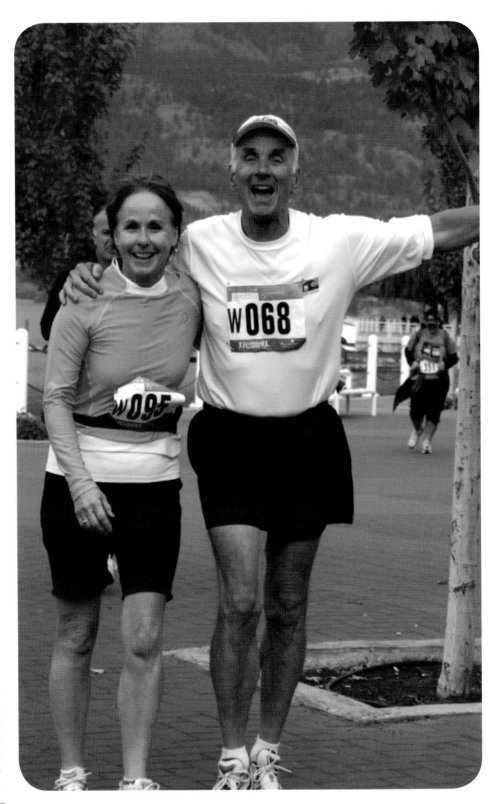

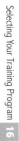

Half Marathon Training - Competitive 2:30:00 (recorded in km)

Week	1	2	3	4	5	6	7	8	9	10	11	12	13	14	15	16	17
Distance Walking	9	20	21	21	23	23	24.5	26	30	34	38.5	40.5	37	42	42	44	25
Walks per Week	3	5	5	5	5	5	5	5	5	5	5	5	5	5	5	5	4

Sample Program

Week	Sun	Mon	Tue	Wed	Thu	Fri	Sat	Weekly Total
1	off	off	off	3 Tempo	3 Steady Walk	off	3 Steady Walk	9
2	7 LSD	off	4 Tempo	3 Tempo	3 Steady Walk	off	3 Steady Walk	20
3	7 LSD	off	4 Tempo	3 Tempo	4 Steady Walk	off	3 Steady Walk	21
4	7 LSD	off	3 Tempo	4 Tempo	3 Steady Walk	off	4 Steady Walk	21
5	9 LSD	off	4 Tempo	4 Tempo	3 Steady Walk	off	3 Steady Walk	23
6	9 LSD	off	5 Tempo	3 Tempo	3 Steady Walk	off	3 Steady Walk	23
7	10 LSD	off	4 Tempo	2.5 3 x 400m Hills	5 Steady Walk	off	3 Steady Walk	24.5
8	10 LSD	off	4 Tempo	3 4 x 400m Hills	5 Steady Walk	off	4 Steady Walk	26
9	12 LSD	off	4 Tempo	4 5 x 400m Hills	6 Steady Walk	off	4 Steady Walk	30
10	14 LSD	off	4 Tempo	5 6 x 400m Hills	6 Steady Walk	off	5 Steady Walk	34
11	16 LSD	off	5 Tempo	5.5 7 x 400m Hills	7 Steady Walk	off	5 Steady Walk	38.5
12	16 LSD	off	5 Tempo	6.5 8 x 400m Hills	7 Steady Walk	off	6 Steady Walk	40.5
13	12 LSD	off	5 Tempo	6 Fartlek	8 Steady Walk	off	6 Steady Walk	37
14	18 LSD	off	6 Tempo	4 Fartlek	8 Steady Walk	off	6 Steady Walk	42
15	18 LSD	off	6 Tempo	4 Fartlek	8 Steady Walk	off	6 Steady Walk	42
16	20 LSD	off	6 Tempo	4 Steady Walk	8 Steady Walk	off	6 Steady Walk	44
17	6 LSD	off	10 Steady Walk	6 Steady Walk	off	off	3 Steady Walk	25
18	21 Race Day							21

Pace Schedule (min/km)

LSD	Steady Pace	Tempo/Hill/Fartlek	Speed	Race Pace	Stroll Adjusted Race Pace
8:03–9:00	8:03	7:17	6:23	7:07	6:53

Pace: LSD & Walk/Stroll Interval = 10 min brisk walk, 1 min relaxed stroll
Hills: Hills are a distance of approximately 400 meters
Snags: If you find any week to be too difficult, repeat that week rather than adding more time, until you are able to progress comfortably.
Pace Breaks: We encourage all walkers to take pace breaks—periods of gentle walking of any kind—as a recovery from the briskness of the periods of effort.

Half Marathon Training - Beginner 3:15:00 (recorded in mi)

Week	1	2	3	4	5	6	7	8	9	10	11	12	13	14	15	16	17
Distance Walking	6	13	13.5	13.5	14.5	15	15	16	18.5	20.5	24	25	22.5	25.5	25.5	27	15
Walks per Week	3	5	5	5	5	5	5	5	5	5	5	5	5	5	5	5	4

Sample Program

Week	Sun	Mon	Tue	Wed	Thu	Fri	Sat	Weekly Total
1	off	off	off	2 Tempo	2 Steady Walk	off	2 Steady Walk	6
2	4.5 LSD	off	2.5 Tempo	2 Tempo	2 Steady Walk	off	2 Steady Walk	13
3	4.5 LSD	off	2.5 Tempo	2 Tempo	2.5 Steady Walk	off	2 Steady Walk	13.5
4	4.5 LSD	off	2 Tempo	2.5 Tempo	2 Steady Walk	off	2.5 Steady Walk	13.5
5	5.5 LSD	off	2.5 Tempo	2.5 Tempo	2 Steady Walk	off	2 Steady Walk	14.5
6	5.5 LSD	off	3 Tempo	2 Tempo	2.5 Steady Walk	off	2 Steady Walk	15
7	6 LSD	off	2.5 Tempo	1.5 3 x 400m Hills	3 Steady Walk	off	2 Steady Walk	15
8	6 LSD	off	2.5 Tempo	2 4 x 400m Hills	3 Steady Walk	off	2.5 Steady Walk	16
9	7.5 LSD	off	2.5 Tempo	2.5 5 x 400m Hills	3.5 Steady Walk	off	2.5 Steady Walk	18.5
10	8.5 LSD	off	2.5 Tempo	3 6 x 400m Hills	3.5 Steady Walk	off	3 Steady Walk	20.5
11	10 LSD	off	3 Tempo	3.5 7 x 400m Hills	4.5 Steady Walk	off	3 Steady Walk	24
12	10 LSD	off	3 Tempo	4 8 x 400m Hills	4.5 Steady Walk	off	3.5 Steady Walk	25
13	7.5 LSD	off	3 Tempo	3.5 Tempo	5 Steady Walk	off	3.5 Steady Walk	22.5
14	11 LSD	off	3.5 Tempo	2.5 Fartlek	5 Steady Walk	off	3.5 Steady Walk	25.5
15	11 LSD	off	3.5 Tempo	2.5 Fartlek	5 Steady Walk	off	3.5 Steady Walk	25.5
16	12.5 LSD	off	3.5 Tempo	2.5 Steady Walk	5 Steady Walk	off	3.5 Steady Walk	27
17	3.5 LSD	off	6 Steady Walk	3.5 Steady Walk	off	off	2 Steady Walk	15
18	13 Race Day							13

Pace Schedule (min/mi)

LSD	Steady Pace	Tempo/Hill/Fartlek	Speed	Race Pace	Stroll Adjusted Race Pace
16:24–18:11	16:24	14:56	13:12	14:52	14:27

Pace: LSD & Walk/Stroll Interval = 10 min brisk walk, 1 min relaxed stroll
Hills: Hills are a distance of approximately 400 meters
Snags: If you find any week to be too difficult, repeat that week rather than adding more time, until you are able to progress comfortably.
Pace Breaks: We encourage all walkers to take pace breaks—periods of gentle walking of any kind—as a recovery from the briskness of the periods of effort.

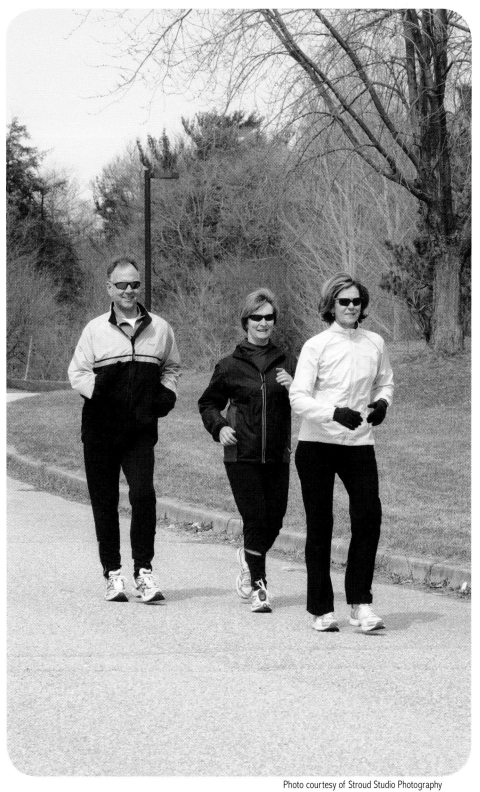

Photo courtesy of Stroud Studio Photography

Half Marathon Training - Intermediate 3:00:00 (recorded in mi)

Week	1	2	3	4	5	6	7	8	9	10	11	12	13	14	15	16	17
Distance Walking	6	13	13.5	13.5	14.5	14.5	15	16	18.5	20.5	24	25	22.5	25.5	25.5	27	15
Walks per Week	3	5	5	5	5	5	5	5	5	5	5	5	5	5	5	5	4

Sample Program

Week	Sun	Mon	Tue	Wed	Thu	Fri	Sat	Weekly Total
1	off	off	off	2 Tempo	2 Steady Walk	off	2 Steady Walk	6
2	4.5 LSD	off	2.5 Tempo	2 Tempo	2 Steady Walk	off	2 Steady Walk	13
3	4.5 LSD	off	2.5 Tempo	2 Tempo	2.5 Steady Walk	off	2 Steady Walk	13.5
4	4.5 LSD	off	2 Tempo	2.5 Tempo	2 Steady Walk	off	2.5 Steady Walk	13.5
5	5.5 LSD	off	2.5 Tempo	2.5 Tempo	2 Steady Walk	off	2 Steady Walk	14.5
6	5.5 LSD	off	3 Tempo	2 Tempo	2 Steady Walk	off	2 Steady Walk	14.5
7	6 LSD	off	2.5 Tempo	1.5 3 x 400m Hills	3 Steady Walk	off	2 Steady Walk	15
8	6 LSD	off	2.5 Tempo	2 4 x 400m Hills	3 Steady Walk	off	2.5 Steady Walk	16
9	7.5 LSD	off	2.5 Tempo	2.5 5 x 400m Hills	3.5 Steady Walk	off	2.5 Steady Walk	18.5
10	8.5 LSD	off	2.5 Tempo	3 6 x 400m Hills	3.5 Steady Walk	off	3 Steady Walk	20.5
11	10 LSD	off	3 Tempo	3.5 7 x 400m Hills	4.5 Steady Walk	off	3 Steady Walk	24
12	10 LSD	off	3 Tempo	4 8 x 400m Hills	4.5 Steady Walk	off	3.5 Steady Walk	25
13	7.5 LSD	off	3 Tempo	3.5 Fartlek	5 Steady Walk	off	3.5 Steady Walk	22.5
14	11 LSD	off	3.5 Tempo	2.5 Fartlek	5 Steady Walk	off	3.5 Steady Walk	25.5
15	11 LSD	off	3.5 Tempo	2.5 Fartlek	5 Steady Walk	off	3.5 Steady Walk	25.5
16	12.5 LSD	off	3.5 Tempo	2.5 Steady Walk	5 Steady Walk	off	3.5 Steady Walk	27
17	3.5 LSD	off	6 Steady Walk	3.5 Active Walking	off	off	2 Steady Walk	15
18	13 Race Day							13

Pace Schedule (min/mi)

LSD	Steady Pace	Tempo/Hill/Fartlek	Speed	Race Pace	Stroll Adjusted Race Pace
15:16–16:58	15:16	13:52	12:13	13:44	13:19

Pace: LSD & Walk/Stroll Interval = 10 min brisk walk, 1 min relaxed stroll
Hills: Hills are a distance of approximately 400 meters
Snags: If you find any week to be too difficult, repeat that week rather than adding more time, until you are able to progress comfortably.
Pace Breaks: We encourage all walkers to take pace breaks—periods of gentle walking of any kind—as a recovery from the briskness of the periods of effort.

Half Marathon Training - Advanced 2:45:00 (recorded in mi)

Week	1	2	3	4	5	6	7	8	9	10	11	12	13	14	15	16	17
Distance Walking	6	13	13.5	13.5	14.5	15	15	16	18.5	20.5	24	24.5	23.5	26.5	25.5	28	15
Walks per Week	3	5	5	5	5	5	5	5	5	5	5	5	5	5	5	5	4

Sample Program

Week	Sun	Mon	Tue	Wed	Thu	Fri	Sat	Weekly Total
1	off	off	off	2 Tempo	2 Steady Walk	off	2 Steady Walk	6
2	4.5 LSD	off	2.5 Tempo	2 Tempo	2 Steady Walk	off	2 Steady Walk	13
3	4.5 LSD	off	2.5 Tempo	2 Tempo	2.5 Steady Walk	off	2 Steady Walk	13.5
4	4.5 LSD	off	2 Tempo	2.5 Tempo	2 Steady Walk	off	2.5 Steady Walk	13.5
5	5.5 LSD	off	2.5 Tempo	2.5 Tempo	2 Steady Walk	off	2 Steady Walk	14.5
6	5.5 LSD	off	3 Tempo	2 Tempo	2.5 Steady Walk	off	2 Steady Walk	15
7	6 LSD	off	2.5 Tempo	1.5 3 x 400m Hills	3 Steady Walk	off	2 Steady Walk	15
8	6 LSD	off	2.5 Tempo	2 4 x 400m Hills	3 Steady Walk	off	2.5 Steady Walk	16
9	7.5 LSD	off	2.5 Tempo	2.5 5 x 400m Hills	3.5 Steady Walk	off	2.5 Steady Walk	18.5
10	8.5 LSD	off	2.5 Tempo	3 6 x 400m Hills	3.5 Steady Walk	off	3 Steady Walk	20.5
11	10 LSD	off	3 Tempo	3.5 7 x 400m Hills	4.5 Steady Walk	off	3 Steady Walk	24
12	10 LSD	off	3 Tempo	4 8 x 400m Hills	4.5 Steady Walk	off	3.5 Steady Walk	25
13	7.5 LSD	off	3 Tempo	4.5 9 x 400m Hills	5 Steady Walk	off	3.5 Steady Walk	23.5
14	11 LSD	off	3.5 Tempo	2.5 Fartlek	5 Steady Walk	off	3.5 Steady Walk	25.5
15	11 LSD	off	3.5 Tempo	2.5 Fartlek	5 Steady Walk	off	3.5 Steady Walk	25.5
16	12.5 LSD	off	3.5 Tempo	2.5 Fartlek	5 Steady Walk	off	3.5 Race Pace	27
17	3.5 LSD	off	6 Steady Walk	3.5 Active Walk	off	off	2 Steady Walk	15
18	13 Race Day							13

Pace Schedule (min/mi)

LSD	Steady Pace	Tempo/Hill/Fartlek	Speed	Race Pace	Stroll Adjusted Race Pace
14:07–15:44	14:07	12:48	11:15	12:35	12:10

Pace: LSD & Walk/Stroll Interval = 10 min brisk walk, 1 min relaxed stroll

Hills: Hills are a distance of approximately 400 meters

Snags: If you find any week to be too difficult, repeat that week rather than adding more time, until you are able to progress comfortably.

Pace Breaks: We encourage all walkers to take pace breaks—periods of gentle walking of any kind—as a recovery from the briskness of the periods of effort.

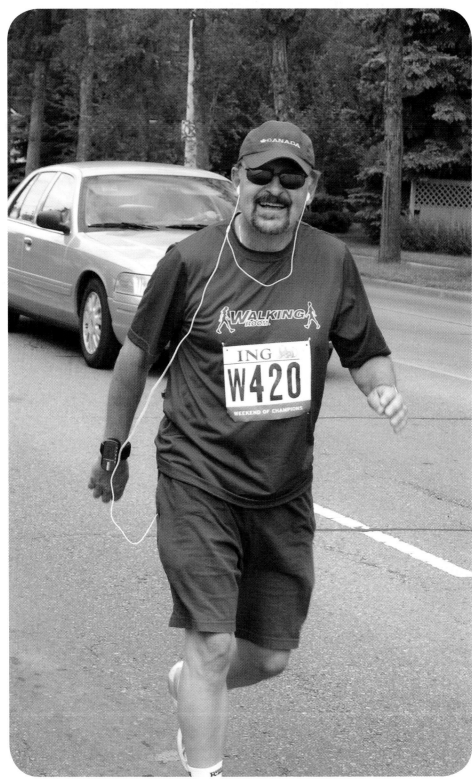

Photo courtesy of tpsphotos.com

Half Marathon Training - Competitive 2:30:00 (recorded in mi)

Week	1	2	3	4	5	6	7	8	9	10	11	12	13	14	15	16	17
Distance Walking	9	20	21	21	23	23	24.5	26	30	34	38.5	40.5	37	42	42	44	25
Walks per Week	3	5	5	5	5	5	5	5	5	5	5	5	5	5	5	5	4

Sample Program

Week	Sun	Mon	Tue	Wed	Thu	Fri	Sat	Weekly Total
1	off	off	off	2 Tempo	2 Steady Walk	off	2 Steady Walk	6
2	4.5 LSD	off	2.5 Tempo	2 Tempo	2 Steady Walk	off	2 Steady Walk	13
3	4.5 LSD	off	2.5 Tempo	2 Tempo	2.5 Steady Walk	off	2 Steady Walk	13.5
4	4.5 LSD	off	2 Tempo	2.5 Tempo	2 Steady Walk	off	2.5 Steady Walk	13.5
5	5.5 LSD	off	2.5 Tempo	2.5 Tempo	2 Steady Walk	off	2 Steady Walk	14.5
6	5.5 LSD	off	3 Tempo	2 Tempo	2 Steady Walk	off	2 Steady Walk	14.5
7	6 LSD	off	2.5 Tempo	1.5 3 x 400m Hills	3 Steady Walk	off	2 Steady Walk	15
8	6 LSD	off	2.5 Tempo	2 4 x 400m Hills	3 Steady Walk	off	2.5 Steady Walk	16
9	7.5 LSD	off	2.5 Tempo	2.5 5 x 400m Hills	3 Steady Walk	off	2.5 Steady Walk	18.5
10	8.5 LSD	off	2.5 Tempo	3 6 x 400m Hills	3.5 Steady Walk	off	3 Steady Walk	20.5
11	10 LSD	off	3 Tempo	3.5 7 x 400m Hills	4.5 Steady Walk	off	3 Steady Walk	24
12	10 LSD	off	3 Tempo	4 8 x 400m Hills	4.5 Steady Walk	off	3.5 Steady Walk	25
13	7.5 LSD	off	3 Tempo	3.5 Fartlek	5 Steady Walk	off	3.5 Steady Walk	22.5
14	11 LSD	off	3.5 Tempo	2.5 Fartlek	5 Steady Walk	off	3.5 Steady Walk	25.5
15	11 LSD	off	3.5 Tempo	2.5 Fartlek	5 Steady Walk	off	3.5 Steady Walk	25.5
16	12.5 LSD	off	3.5 Tempo	2.5 Fartlek	5 Steady Walk	off	3.5 Steady Walk	27
17	3.5 LSD	off	6 Steady Walk	3.5 Active Walking	off	off	2 Steady Walk	15
18	13 Race Day							13

Pace Schedule (min/mi)

LSD	Steady Pace	Tempo/Hill/Fartlek	Speed	Race Pace	Stroll Adjusted Race Pace
12:57–14:29	12:57	11:43	10:16	11:27	11:02

Pace: LSD & Walk/Stroll Interval = 10 min brisk walk, 1 min relaxed stroll
Hills: Hills are a distance of approximately 400 meters
Snags: If you find any week to be too difficult, repeat that week rather than adding more time, until you are able to progress comfortably.
Pace Breaks: We encourage all walkers to take pace breaks—periods of gentle walking of any kind—as a recovery from the briskness of the periods of effort.

16 Selecting Your Training Program

Marathon Walking Programs

The Marathon

Are you ready for the ultimate walking challenge? You'll find it in the marathon.

Training for the marathon can positively change the way you look at the rest of your life: you will experience a dramatic change in your physical and mental outlook on life and you will gain the self-confidence to achieve both your athletic and personal goals. By training to walk a marathon, you'll find personal resources you didn't know were there.

The largest-growing group in the modern marathon is composed of people who just want to complete the 42.2-km (26.2-mi) course. Over the years it has become obvious that not all of us can be competitive marathoners. Just as our fingerprints are unique to each of us, so are our other attributes, such as body type, resting heart rate, maximum heart rate and requirements put on us by family, work, friends and commitments to the community.

If you decide the marathon is your event, don't plan on doing more than two in a year. This gives you lots of time to rest, recover and start training for the next race.

Selecting a Program

On the following pages you will find a variety of suggested training schedules. These schedules have been designed to help walkers complete the event and achieve specific time goals. The programs all follow the progressive structure as outlined in *Chapter 4—Developing Your Walking Program*. Long walks incorporate the 10/1 walk/stroll (stress and rest) principle that has made my programs so successful. In addition, you will see at the bottom of every training schedule a pace chart outlining the pace requirements for each walk. Below you will find a description of the various types of workouts as reflected in the training schedules. You can refer to *Chapter 4—Developing Your Walking Program* for a more detailed description of training methods. In addition *Chapter 3—Training Concepts & Terms* provides a nice review of the various workout requirements of a successful walking program.

Tapering for a Marathon

Many experienced marathoner walkers will tell you that you'll only perform as well as you've tapered. Many people forget that training is hard work and you can't just jump into an event and perform well without proper planning. Everyone's performance can benefit from a good taper, which is a carefully planned period of reduced training. This gradual easing up allows your body to disperse the residual fatigue products carried from one workout to another. The extra recovery and regeneration occurring as a result of a taper is called peaking. Come race day, your legs will have that extra snap to ensure your best performance.

The biggest complaint about tapering is people often feel extremely restless during this period—they feel like they should be doing more. Please don't. The beginning of the taper period signifies the end of training and the beginning of competition preparation. Any hard training done during this period will do more to hurt your performance than help it because you won't recover fast enough. A good taper will make you feel like a horse in the gate at the start of the race for the few days before your event. This is the feeling of peak fitness; use it to your advantage.

A taper for a marathon should generally take up the last two to three weeks before the event. Your last long walk should take place no later than two weeks before the event. During the taper period, you should walk only 30–50% of your regular weekly distance. The best tapers have walkers maintaining their training intensity while gradually reducing their training distance to practically zero a few days before the event. Focus on keeping the intensity up on your continuous walks and reducing their length significantly. Forget speed training if you have any planned.

Your last quality workout should be on the second Saturday before the race. Walk 16 km (10 mi) at your target pace for the marathon. This walk is a high-quality workout that requires your discipline, so it is best to walk it alone and concentrate on your form and setting the targeted pace. Do not race or get in a race with one of your training partners. Work at your race pace and include your walking 10 minutes/strolling 1 minute combinations. Starting on Monday, you will begin to cut back your distance in the tapering phase of the program. Some people feel very heavy and their disposition suffers during the tapering phase. Concentrate on the joy of less distance and the fact that you have all this extra time to relax and enjoy the tapering phase.

The most important day is two days prior to the race. Take the day off, go to bed early and enjoy as much sleep as possible. Stay in bed, read and relax. Even if you can't sleep, stay lying down. It's the best way to get you ready for race day. Remember, nothing you do in the final week will help you, but everything you do can hinder your performance. Quality training takes at least two weeks to improve your performance, but overtraining can affect your performance the next day.

Visualization is a key part of the week as you relax and think about your training and the goals you have set for the marathon. Read or listen to some of your favorite music to motivate yourself.

Marathon Training Programs (recorded in Km)

Marathon Training Programs (recorded in mi)

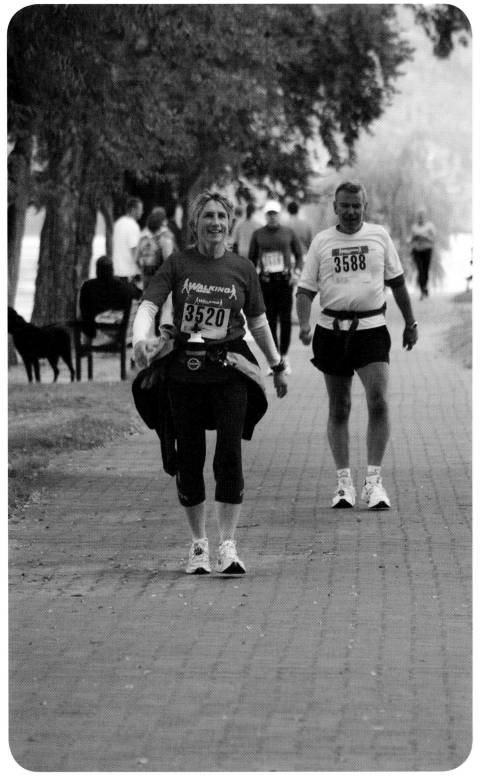

Marathon Training - Beginner 6:30:00 (recorded in km)

Week	1	2	3	4	5	6	7	8	9	10	11	12	13	14	15	16	17	18
Distance Walking	38	38	43	43	46	46	44	51	55	49.5	60.5	62	66	55	61	64	55	25
Walks per Week	5	5	5	5	5	5	5	5	5	5	5	5	5	5	5	5	5	4

Sample Program

Week	Sun	Mon	Tue	Wed	Thu	Fri	Sat	Weekly Total
1	10 LSD	off	6 Tempo	10 Tempo	6 Steady Walk	off	6 Steady Walk	38
2	10 LSD	off	6 Tempo	10 Tempo	6 Steady Walk	off	6 Steady Walk	38
3	13 LSD	off	6 Tempo	10 Tempo	8 Steady Walk	off	6 Steady Walk	43
4	13 LSD	off	6 Tempo	10 Tempo	8 Steady Walk	off	6 Steady Walk	43
5	16 LSD	off	6 Tempo	10 Tempo	8 Steady Walk	off	6 Steady Walk	46
6	16 LSD	off	6 Tempo	10 Tempo	8 Steady Walk	off	6 Steady Walk	46
7	19 LSD	off	6 Tempo	5 4 x 600m Hills	8 Steady Walk	off	6 Steady Walk	44
8	23 LSD	off	6 Tempo	6 5 x 600m Hills	10 Steady Walk	off	6 Steady Walk	51
9	26 LSD	off	6 Tempo	7 6 x 600m Hills	10 Steady Walk	off	6 Steady Walk	55
10	19 LSD	off	6 Tempo	8.5 7 x 600m Hills	10 Steady Walk	off	6 Steady Walk	49.5
11	29 LSD	off	6 Tempo	9.5 8 x 600m Hills	10 Steady Walk	off	6 Steady Walk	60.5
12	29 LSD	off	6 Tempo	11 9 x 600m Hills	10 Steady Walk	off	6 Steady Walk	62
13	32 LSD	off	6 Tempo	12 10 x 600m Hills	10 Steady Walk	off	6 Steady Walk	66
14	23 LSD	off	6 Tempo	10 Fartlek	10 Steady Walk	off	6 Steady Walk	55
15	29 LSD	off	6 Tempo	10 Fartlek	10 Steady Walk	off	6 Steady Walk	61
16	32 LSD	off	6 Tempo	10 Fartlek	10 Steady Walk	off	6 Steady Walk	64
17	23 LSD	off	6 Tempo	10 Fartlek	10 Steady Walk	off	6 Steady Walk	55
18	6 LSD	off	6 Tempo	10 Active Walking	off	off	3 Steady Walk	25
19	42 Race Day							42

Pace Schedule (min/km)

LSD	Steady Pace	Tempo/Hill/Fartlek	Speed	Race Pace	Stroll Adjusted Race Pace
10:04–11:10	10:04	9:10	8:06	9:15	9:06

Pace: LSD & Walk/Stroll Interval = 10 min brisk walk, 1 min relaxed stroll

Hills: Hills are a distance of approximately 600 meters

Snags: If you find any week to be too difficult, repeat that week, rather than adding more time, until you are able to progress comfortably.

Pace Breaks: We encourage all walkers to take pace breaks—periods of gentle walking of any kind—as a recovery from the briskness of the periods of effort.

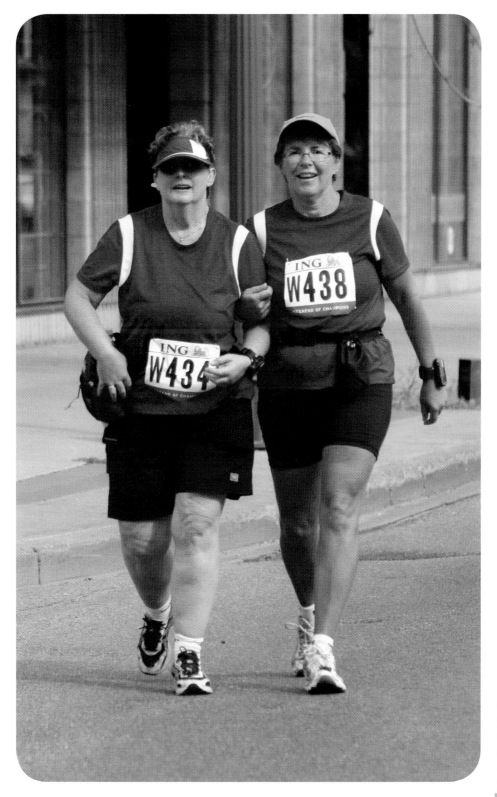

Marathon Training - Intermediate 6:00:00 (recorded in km)

Week	1	2	3	4	5	6	7	8	9	10	11	12	13	14	15	16	17	18
Distance Walking	38	38	43	43	46	46	44	51	55	49.5	60.5	62	66	55	61	64	55	25
Walks per Week	5	5	5	5	5	5	5	5	5	5	5	5	5	5	5	5	5	4

Sample Program

Week	Sun	Mon	Tue	Wed	Thu	Fri	Sat	Weekly Total
1	10 LSD	off	6 Tempo	10 Tempo	6 Steady Walk	off	6 Steady Walk	38
2	10 LSD	off	6 Tempo	10 Tempo	6 Steady Walk	off	6 Steady Walk	38
3	13 LSD	off	6 Tempo	10 Tempo	8 Steady Walk	off	6 Steady Walk	43
4	13 LSD	off	6 Tempo	10 Tempo	8 Steady Walk	off	6 Steady Walk	43
5	16 LSD	off	6 Tempo	10 Tempo	8 Steady Walk	off	6 Steady Walk	46
6	16 LSD	off	6 Tempo	10 Tempo	8 Steady Walk	off	6 Steady Walk	46
7	19 LSD	off	6 Tempo	5 4 x 600m Hills	8 Steady Walk	6 Steady Walk	off	44
8	23 LSD	off	6 Tempo	6 5 x 600m Hills	10 Steady Walk	off	6 Steady Walk	51
9	26 LSD	off	6 Tempo	7 6 x 600m Hills	10 Steady Walk	off	6 Steady Walk	55
10	19 LSD	off	6 Tempo	8.5 7 x 600m Hills	10 Steady Walk	off	6 Steady Walk	49.5
11	29 LSD	off	6 Tempo	9.5 8 x 600m Hills	10 Steady Walk	off	6 Steady Walk	60.5
12	29 LSD	off	6 Tempo	11 9 x 600m Hills	10 Steady Walk	off	6 Steady Walk	62
13	32 LSD	off	6 Tempo	12 10 x 600m Hills	10 Steady Walk	off	6 Steady Walk	66
14	23 LSD	off	6 Tempo	10 Fartlek	10 Steady Walk	off	6 Steady Walk	55
15	29 LSD	off	6 Tempo	10 Fartlek	10 Steady Walk	off	6 Steady Walk	61
16	32 LSD	off	6 Tempo	10 Fartlek	10 Steady Walk	off	6 Steady Walk	64
17	23 LSD	off	6 Tempo	10 Fartlek	10 Steady Walk	off	6 Steady Walk	55
18	6 LSD	off	6 Tempo	10 Active Walking	off	off	3 Steady Walk	25
19	42 Race Day							42

Pace Schedule (min/km)

LSD	Steady Pace	Tempo/Hill/Fartlek	Speed	Race Pace	Stroll Adjusted Race Pace
9:21–10:24	9:21	8:29	7:28	8:32	8:21

Pace: LSD & Walk/Stroll Interval = 10 min brisk walk, 1 min relaxed stroll
Hills: Hills are a distance of approximately 600 meters
Snags: If you find any week to be too difficult, repeat that week, rather than adding more time, until you are able to progress comfortably.
Pace Breaks: We encourage all walkers to take pace breaks——periods of gentle walking of any kind——as a recovery from the briskness of the periods of effort.

Marathon Training - Advanced 5:45:00 (recorded in km)

Week	1	2	3	4	5	6	7	8	9	10	11	12	13	14	15	16	17	18
Distance Walking	38	38	43	43	46	46	44	51	55	49.5	60.5	62	66	55	61	64	55	25
Walks per Week	5	5	5	5	5	5	5	5	5	5	5	5	5	5	5	5	5	4

Sample Program

Week	Sun	Mon	Tue	Wed	Thu	Fri	Sat	Weekly Total
1	10 LSD	off	6 Tempo	10 Tempo	6 Steady Walk	off	6 Steady Walk	38
2	10 LSD	off	6 Tempo	10 Tempo	6 Steady Walk	off	6 Steady Walk	38
3	13 LSD	off	6 Tempo	10 Tempo	8 Steady Walk	off	6 Steady Walk	43
4	13 LSD	off	6 Tempo	10 Tempo	8 Steady Walk	off	6 Steady Walk	43
5	16 LSD	off	6 Tempo	10 Tempo	8 Steady Walk	off	6 Steady Walk	46
6	16 LSD	off	6 Tempo	10 Tempo	8 Steady Walk	off	6 Steady Walk	46
7	19 LSD	off	6 Tempo	5 4 x 600m Hills	8 Steady Walk	off	6 Steady Walk	44
8	23 LSD	off	6 Tempo	6 5 x 600m Hills	10 Steady Walk	off	6 Steady Walk	51
9	26 LSD	off	6 Tempo	7 6 x 600m Hills	10 Steady Walk	off	6 Steady Walk	55
10	19 LSD	off	6 Tempo	8.5 7 x 600m Hills	10 Steady Walk	off	6 Steady Walk	49.5
11	29 LSD	off	6 Tempo	9.5 8 x 600m Hills	10 Steady Walk	off	6 Steady Walk	60.5
12	29 LSD	off	6 Tempo	11 9 x 600m Hills	10 Steady Walk	off	6 Steady Walk	62
13	32 LSD	off	6 Tempo	12 10 x 600m Hills	10 Steady Walk	off	6 Steady Walk	66
14	23 LSD	off	6 Tempo	10 Fartlek	10 Steady Walk	off	6 Steady Walk	55
15	29 LSD	off	6 Tempo	10 Fartlek	10 Steady Walk	off	6 Steady Walk	61
16	32 LSD	off	6 Tempo	10 Fartlek	10 Steady Walk	off	6 Steady Walk	64
17	23 LSD	off	6 Tempo	10 Fartlek	10 Steady Walk	off	6 Steady Walk	55
18	6 LSD	off	6 Tempo	10 Active Walking	off	off	3 Steady Walk	25
19	42 Race Day							42

Pace Schedule (min/km)

LSD	Steady Pace	Tempo/Hill/Fartlek	Speed	Race Pace	Stroll Adjusted Race Pace
8:59–10:00	8:59	8:09	7:10	8:11	7:59

Pace: LSD & Walk/Stroll Interval = 10 min brisk walk, 1 min relaxed stroll
Hills: Hills are a distance of approximately 600 meters
Snags: If you find any week to be too difficult, repeat that week, rather than adding more time, until you are able to progress comfortably.
Pace Breaks: We encourage all walkers to take pace breaks—periods of gentle walking of any kind—as a recovery from the briskness of the periods of effort.

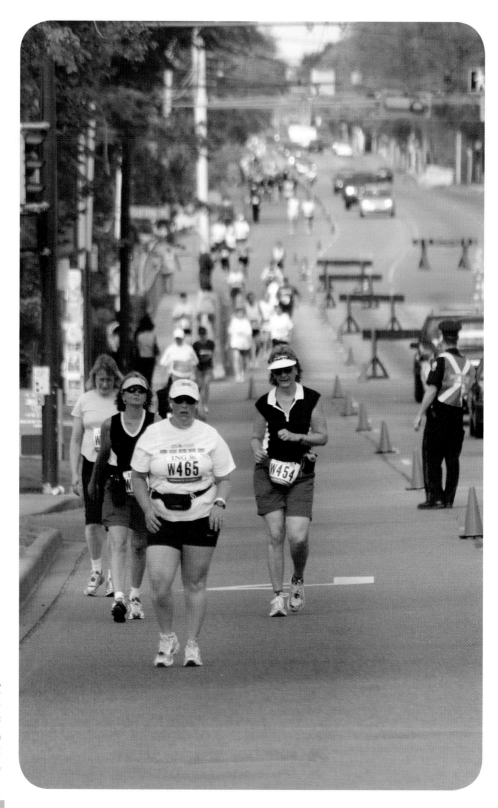

Marathon Training - Beginner 6:30:00 (recorded in mi)

Week	1	2	3	4	5	6	7	8	9	10	11	12	13	14	15	16	17	18
Distance Walking	22.5	22.5	26	26	28	28	27	31	33.5	30	37	37.5	40.5	33.5	37	39	33.5	15
Walks per Week	5	5	5	5	5	5	5	5	5	5	5	5	5	5	5	5	5	4

Sample Program

Week	Sun	Mon	Tue	Wed	Thu	Fri	Sat	Weekly Total
1	6 LSD	off	3.5 Tempo	6 Tempo	3.5 Steady Walk	off	3.5 Steady Walk	22.5
2	6 LSD	off	3.5 Tempo	6 Tempo	3.5 Steady Walk	off	3.5 Steady Walk	22.5
3	8 LSD	off	3.5 Tempo	6 Tempo	5 Steady Walk	off	3.5 Steady Walk	26
4	8 LSD	off	3.5 Tempo	6 Tempo	5 Steady Walk	off	3.5 Steady Walk	26
5	10 LSD	off	3.5 Tempo	6 Tempo	5 Steady Walk	off	3.5 Steady Walk	28
6	10 LSD	off	3.5 Tempo	6 Tempo	5 Steady Walk	off	3.5 Steady Walk	28
7	12 LSD	off	3.5 Tempo	3 4 x 600m Hills	5 Steady Walk	off	3.5 Steady Walk	27
8	14.5 LSD	off	3.5 Tempo	3.5 5 x 600m Hills	6 Steady Walk	off	3.5 Steady Walk	31
9	16 LSD	off	3.5 Tempo	4.5 6 x 600m Hills	6 Steady Walk	off	3.5 Steady Walk	33.5
10	12 LSD	off	3.5 Tempo	5 7 x 600m Hills	6 Steady Walk	off	3.5 Steady Walk	30
11	18 LSD	off	3.5 Tempo	6 8 x 600m Hills	6 Steady Walk	off	3.5 Steady Walk	37
12	18 LSD	off	3.5 Tempo	6.5 9 x 600m Hills	6 Steady Walk	off	3.5 Steady Walk	37.5
13	20 LSD	off	3.5 Tempo	7.5 10 x 600m Hills	6 Steady Walk	off	3.5 Steady Walk	40.5
14	14.5 LSD	off	3.5 Tempo	6 Fartlek	6 Steady Walk	off	3.5 Steady Walk	33.5
15	18 LSD	off	3.5 Tempo	6 Fartlek	6 Steady Walk	off	3.5 Steady Walk	37
16	20 LSD	off	3.5 Tempo	6 Fartlek	6 Steady Walk	off	3.5 Steady Walk	39
17	14.5 LSD	off	3.5 Tempo	6 Fartlek	6 Steady Walk	off	3.5 Steady Walk	33.5
18	3.5 LSD	off	3.5 Tempo	6 Active Walking	off	off	2 Steady Walk	15
19	26 Race Day							26

Pace Schedule (min/km)

LSD	Steady Pace	Tempo/Hill/Fartlek	Speed	Race Pace	Stroll Adjusted Race Pace
16:12–17:58	16:12	14:45	13:01	14:52	14:27

Pace: LSD & Walk/Stroll Interval = 10 min brisk walk, 1 min relaxed stroll
Hills: Hills are a distance of approximately 600 meters
Snags: If you find any week to be too difficult, repeat that week, rather than adding more time, until you are able to progress comfortably.
Pace Breaks: We encourage all walkers to take pace breaks—periods of gentle walking of any kind—as a recovery from the briskness of the periods of effort.

16 Selecting Your Training Program

Marathon Training - Intermediate 6:00:00 (recorded in mi)

Week	1	2	3	4	5	6	7	8	9	10	11	12	13	14	15	16	17	18
Distance Walking	22.5	22.5	26	26	28	28	27	31	33.5	30	37	37.5	40.5	33.5	37	39	33.5	15
Walks per Week	5	5	5	5	5	5	5	5	5	5	5	5	5	5	5	5	5	4

Sample Program

Week	Sun	Mon	Tue	Wed	Thu	Fri	Sat	Weekly Total
1	6 LSD	off	3.5 Tempo	6 Tempo	3.5 Steady Walk	off	3.5 Steady Walk	22.5
2	6 LSD	off	3.5 Tempo	6 Tempo	3.5 Steady Walk	off	3.5 Steady Walk	22.5
3	8 LSD	off	3.5 Tempo	6 Tempo	5 Steady Walk	off	3.5 Steady Walk	26
4	8 LSD	off	3.5 Tempo	6 Tempo	5 Steady Walk	off	3.5 Steady Walk	26
5	10 LSD	off	3.5 Tempo	6 Tempo	5 Steady Walk	off	3.5 Steady Walk	28
6	10 LSD	off	3.5 Tempo	6 Tempo	5 Steady Walk	off	3.5 Steady Walk	28
7	12 LSD	off	3.5 Tempo	3 4 x 600m Hills	5 Steady Walk	3.5 Steady Walk	off	27
8	14.5 LSD	off	3.5 Tempo	3.5 5 x 600m Hills	6 Steady Walk	off	3.5 Steady Walk	31
9	16 LSD	off	3.5 Tempo	4.5 6 x 600m Hills	6 Steady Walk	off	3.5 Steady Walk	33.5
10	12 LSD	off	3.5 Tempo	5 7 x 600m Hills	6 Steady Walk	off	3.5 Steady Walk	30
11	18 LSD	off	3.5 Tempo	6 8 x 600m Hills	6 Steady Walk	off	3.5 Steady Walk	37
12	18 LSD	off	3.5 Tempo	6.5 9 x 600m Hills	6 Steady Walk	off	3.5 Steady Walk	37.5
13	20 LSD	off	3.5 Tempo	7.5 10 x 600m Hills	6 Steady Walk	off	3.5 Steady Walk	40.5
14	14.5 LSD	off	3.5 Tempo	6 Fartlek	6 Steady Walk	off	3.5 Steady Walk	33.5
15	18 LSD	off	3.5 Tempo	6 Fartlek	6 Steady Walk	off	3.5 Steady Walk	37
16	20 LSD	off	3.5 Tempo	6 Fartlek	6 Steady Walk	off	3.5 Steady Walk	39
17	14.5 LSD	off	3.5 Tempo	6 Fartlek	6 Steady Walk	off	3.5 Steady Walk	33.5
18	3.5 LSD	off	3.5 Tempo	6 Active Walking	off	off	2 Steady Walk	15
19	26 Race Day							26

Pace Schedule (min/km)

LSD	Steady Pace	Tempo/Hill/Fartlek	Speed	Race Pace	Stroll Adjusted Race Pace
15:02–16:44	15:02	13:40	12:02	13:44	13:19

Pace: LSD & Walk/Stroll Interval = 10 min brisk walk, 1 min relaxed stroll

Hills: Hills are a distance of approximately 600 meters

Snags: If you find any week to be too difficult, repeat that week, rather than adding more time, until you are able to progress comfortably.

Pace Breaks: We encourage all walkers to take pace breaks—periods of gentle walking of any kind—as a recovery from the briskness of the periods of effort.

Marathon Training - Advanced 5:45:00 (recorded in mi)

Week	1	2	3	4	5	6	7	8	9	10	11	12	13	14	15	16	17	18
Distance Walking	22.5	22.5	26	26	28	28	27	31	33.5	30	37	37.5	40.5	33.5	37	39	33.5	15
Walks per Week	5	5	5	5	5	5	5	5	5	5	5	5	5	5	5	5	5	4

Sample Program

Week	Sun	Mon	Tue	Wed	Thu	Fri	Sat	Weekly Total
1	6 LSD	off	3.5 Tempo	6 Tempo	3.5 Steady Walk	off	3.5 Steady Walk	22.5
2	6 LSD	off	3.5 Tempo	6 Tempo	3.5 Steady Walk	off	3.5 Steady Walk	22.5
3	8 LSD	off	3.5 Tempo	6 Tempo	5 Steady Walk	off	3.5 Steady Walk	26
4	8 LSD	off	3.5 Tempo	6 Tempo	5 Steady Walk	off	3.5 Steady Walk	26
5	10 LSD	off	3.5 Tempo	6 Tempo	5 Steady Walk	off	3.5 Steady Walk	28
6	10 LSD	off	3.5 Tempo	6 Tempo	5 Steady Walk	off	3.5 Steady Walk	28
7	12 LSD	off	3.5 Tempo	3 4 x 600m Hills	5 Steady Walk	off	3.5 Steady Walk	27
8	14.5 LSD	off	3.5 Tempo	3.5 5 x 600m Hills	6 Steady Walk	off	3.5 Steady Walk	31
9	16 LSD	off	3.5 Tempo	4.5 6 x 600m Hills	6 Steady Walk	off	3.5 Steady Walk	33.5
10	12 LSD	off	3.5 Tempo	5 7 x 600m Hills	6 Steady Walk	off	3.5 Steady Walk	30
11	18 LSD	off	3.5 Tempo	6 8 x 600m Hills	6 Steady Walk	off	3.5 Steady Walk	37
12	18 LSD	off	3.5 Tempo	6.5 9 x 600m Hills	6 Steady Walk	off	3.5 Steady Walk	37.5
13	20 LSD	off	3.5 Tempo	7.5 10 x 600m Hills	6 Steady Walk	off	3.5 Steady Walk	40.5
14	14.5 LSD	off	3.5 Tempo	6 Fartlek	6 Steady Walk	off	3.5 Steady Walk	33.5
15	18 LSD	off	3.5 Tempo	6 Fartlek	6 Steady Walk	off	3.5 Steady Walk	37
16	20 LSD	off	3.5 Tempo	6 Fartlek	6 Steady Walk	off	3.5 Steady Walk	39
17	14.5 LSD	off	3.5 Tempo	6 Fartlek	6 Steady Walk	off	3.5 Steady Walk	33.5
18	3.5 LSD	off	3.5 Tempo	6 Active Walking	off	off	2 Steady Walk	15
19	26 Race Day							26

Pace Schedule (min/km)

LSD	Steady Pace	Tempo/Hill/Fartlek	Speed	Race Pace	Stroll Adjusted Race Pace
14:27–16:06	14:27	13:07	11:32	13:10	12:45

Pace: LSD & Walk/Stroll Interval = 10 min brisk walk, 1 min relaxed stroll
Hills: Hills are a distance of approximately 600 meters
Snags: If you find any week to be too difficult, repeat that week, rather than adding more time, until you are able to progress comfortably.
Pace Breaks: We encourage all walkers to take pace breaks—periods of gentle walking of any kind—as a recovery from the briskness of the periods of effort.

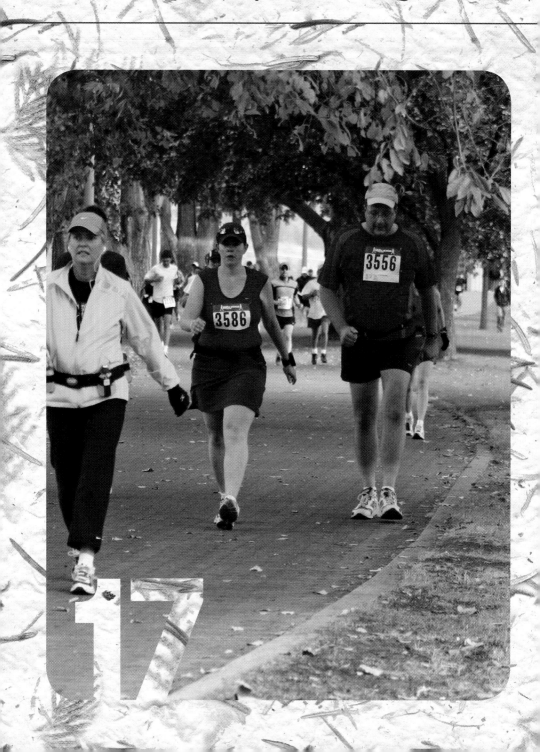

17

Most Frequently Asked Questions

For easy reference, we've compiled what we have found to be some of the most common questions posted to our website. We have edited some of the original text for clarity.

You will see from the following responses that we rely on the knowledge base of our network of professionals in response to questions requiring a level of expertise in their specific discipline. There are certain areas of expertise best left to heath care professionals. We are fortunate to be associated with many illustrious professionals in the areas of medicine, sports training, nutrition and sports injury. We acknowledge their input and thank them for the comprehensive advice they give to ensure our readers get the proper information.

Visit our website:

www.runningroom.com (it is a valuable source of information).

What's a heart rate monitor?

It consists of a watch worn on your wrist and a transmitter that you comfortably wear against your skin and around your chest. The transmitter picks up the signals of your heart, and sends them wirelessly to the watch you wear on your wrist. It's that simple. No wires, no stopping to take your pulse and doing a multiplication equation. Just look at your wrist and it's there. The continuous display is what makes it effective. The monitor is your silent coach, guiding you during your workout. Heart rate monitors are reliable and easy to use.

—John Stanton

What are the symptoms of heat exhaustion?

They are loss of concentration, hot and cold flashes, clammy skin, you have stopped sweating, nausea, rapid build-up of heat in the head, goosebumps and slurred speech.

—John Stanton

Many walkers make a cup of coffee a part of their pre-walk/pre-race routine. But what effect does caffeine really have on performance?

There are several ways caffeine may improve performance in endurance events. Caffeine stimulates the central nervous system that facilitates neuromuscular function by improving muscle contraction/reaction time. This effect on the CNS may also lead to a decreased perception of fatigue.

Another potentially beneficial effect of caffeine for walkers is an increased concentration of free fatty acids in the blood and increased uptake and utilization of these fatty acids by muscle tissue. This, in turn, spares the muscles' limited supply of glycogen. The importance of this effect is illustrated by the term "hitting the wall," which is the point at which a person's glycogen stores have been completely depleted.

All of this makes caffeine sound like it's the ultimate aid for the long distance athlete. However, there is a downside to the use of caffeine.

The first is that caffeine is a potent diuretic. Staying well hydrated is one of the keys to quality walks in training and competition. Therefore, ensure that you increase your fluid intake if you are going to take caffeine prior to working out. Caffeine also increases the secretion of acid into the stomach, which can lead to cramps and stomach pain—definitely two things you don't need in the middle of a long walk.

Before you decide whether or not caffeine is for you, there are a few other factors to consider. One is that tolerance is easily built up. Therefore, the effect that caffeine may have on your performance will be limited if you are a regular coffee, cola or tea drinker. So give yourself two or three caffeine-free days before trying it out in your program. As well, like all other changes to your walking program, try it out first in training and not in competition.

If you do decide to use caffeine, the optimum dose for positive effects is 2–3 mg/kg of body weight. (There are about 80 mg in a cup of brewed coffee and 40 mg in a can of Coke.) The effects of caffeine peak around 30 minutes after ingestion and continue for two to three hours.

Armed with some facts, you can now decide what's best for you!
—John Stanton

I've always had a strong desire to fitness walk and when I've walked in the past I have always gotten a rush from doing so. It's a great stress reliever. The unfortunate thing and the source of many of my problems is that I have to quit smoking before I can start fitness walking again. Any suggestions? I know that question may sound corny in this day and age of pills, patches, hypnotism, etc., but I just thought you guys, since you have a well organized club may have a few secrets that everyone can benefit from.

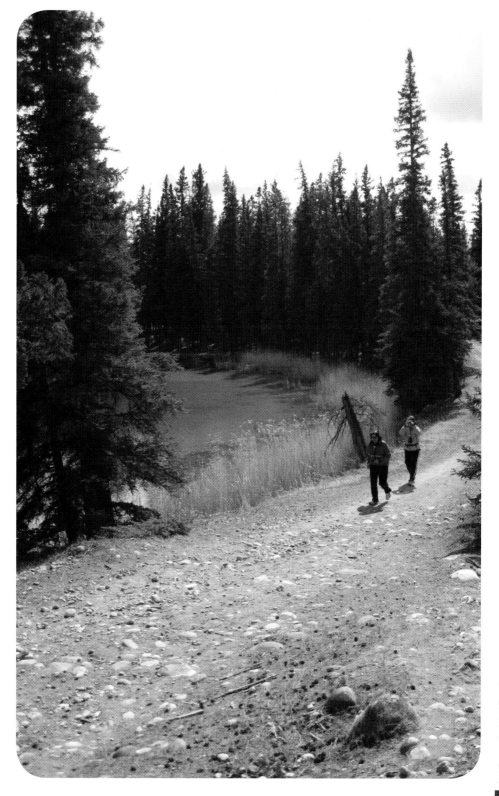

This may sound silly, but for the time being do not try to stop smoking cold turkey. You are much better off substituting a positive addiction for a negative one. Try 20 minutes of brisk walk/strolling combinations, incorporating brisk walking for one minute/strolling for one minute. Start with every second day. Each week add an additional one minute of walking to each walking set. As an example, in week 2 you will brisk walk for two minutes and stroll for one minute. As you progress each week and see the benefits of the exercise you will find the self-motivation to cut back or quit smoking totally. This personal commitment and decision is a much more powerful change of focus and self-improvement than a patch. Seeing our improvement in appearance and self-esteem drives home the lifestyle change. Walking has a number of marvelous benefits to one's personal life. It's a great stress buster, calorie burner and in addition walking with a buddy can be very social. Keep your walking and changes that you make fun and positive. Depravation usually only sets up the urge and desire for the very thing we are trying to do without. A positive change initiates the lifestyle adjustment long term. You can do this. Try the walking and enjoy the improvements to the quality of your life. Above all have fun! Think of your new addition as play.
—John Stanton

Why do I hurt more now after my workouts than I used to? I am 50 years old. Is it something I just have to "grin and bear"?

There are many reasons that you hurt after training. The more obvious ones include training errors, repetitive stress syndromes, lactic acid retention, improper footwear and anatomical conditions. In the above question, the writer implied it might have been his/her age. Aging is simply the process of growing older. (How can aging be simple?) It describes the progressive changes produced by the passage of time. During this time we might expect to see our endurance decrease, our race times slow, our injuries increase and the time to heal them increase. It should not be a time to dwell on how fast or how strong we were several decades ago. Our enjoyment of the sport should continue to increase, and in order to ensure this, some adaptations to our sport must be made. Our expectations of why we are active have to be prioritized. What if our enjoyment doesn't meet our expectations? Why do some athletes at an older age experience more pain and aches when they are active?

Are we supposed to get hurt physically and mentally as we walk into the sunset? The answer to this is a categorical NO!
To address these issues it is important to understand some basic physiology.

The human body is composed of several organ systems, various tissues and many cells. It is these cells that are responsible for the production of energy to make muscles and other tissues work. As we mature, the various relationships between the cellular elements change. The elasticity of the skin, muscle and other organs diminishes and is replaced with fibrous tissue and fat. Neither of these tissues is particularly suited to movement and stretching, so we can expect to see a decrease in flexibility of the joints, muscles and tendons with increasing age. This lack of flexibility is probably the most important factor in decreasing muscle output and increasing injury occurrence with age. The lack of muscle flexibility results in poorer muscle contractions in the heart and hence reduced cardiac output. This will result in a decreased VO2 Max.

—John Stanton

Why does VO2 Max decrease with age?

A Word on VO2 Max

In exercise, an increase in oxygen consumption follows an increase in exercise intensity. The point at which the athlete can take in or use no more oxygen is the point of maximum oxygen consumption. VO2 Max is the maximum rate of oxygen flow and usually is expressed relative to body weight (e.g., ml/kg/min.).

Healthy persons experience a gradual decrease in VO2 Max by approximately 10% per decade after 25 years of age. In prime athletes this reduction may be only 5% per decade.

1. There is a decrease in heart rate with age and therefore a decrease in cardiac output.

2. There may be a decrease in muscle contraction or a loss of muscle mass with age.

Speed deteriorates faster with increasing age than does endurance. Peak performance in marathons, for example, occurs in the range of 25–30 years. After

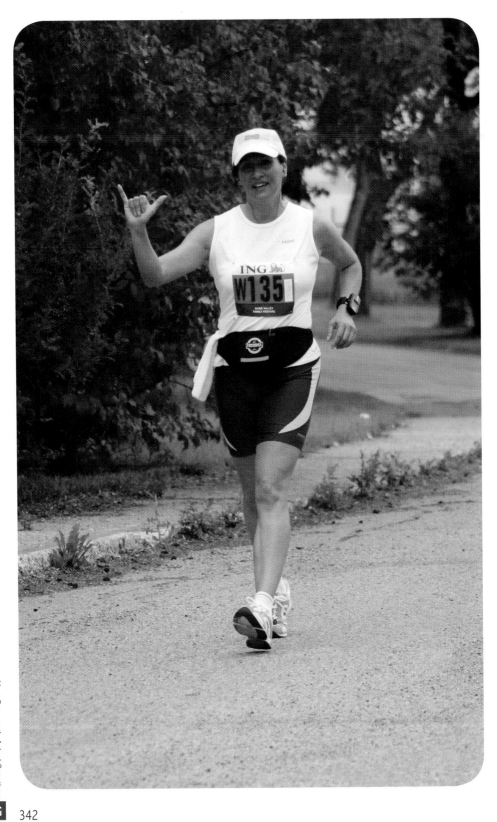

40 years of age there is a linear decline in performance. This fall in performance mirrors a fall in an athlete's VO2 Max.

Therefore, there are definite reasons why, as we age, we are slower and possibly get injured more frequently. As a "master" athlete you have to realize this normal physiological phenomenon and adjust your walking accordingly. We are no longer the flexible, muscular gazelles we once were. Our walking times are slower. Our limbs are not as flexible—they're stiffer. Our muscles are weaker. We are more prone to minor injuries and in some situations more prone to major injuries. But it is important for a number of reasons to keep active: cardiovascular (there is a reduced death rate from heart attacks in athletes); musculoskeletal (there is a decreased incidence of osteoporosis in recreational athletes); and psychological (there is less depression in athletes and those who keep active).

In this particular case, the questioner would have to look at his or her walking program. Stroll breaks are especially important for the older athletes. Keep hydrating. Recovery time is equally important; therefore, rest after a walk. Doing tempo walks too close together will result in increased injuries and increased pain. Pre- and post-walk stretches are important but not always necessary for your short walks.

Research indicates that athletes who remain fit can expect a 0.5–1% decline in performance per year from age 35 to 60. After age 60, performance decline tends to be at a faster rate. On the positive side, appropriate training tends to decrease this performance decline compared to inactive seniors. A study described in the *British Journal of Sports Medicine* (August 2004) showed that after analyzing 415,000 athletes in the New York City Marathon from 1983 to 1999, male and female masters continued to improve times at a greater rate than the younger athletes, whose performance levels had reached a plateau!

Many athletes continue to run or walk into their 60s and 70s and beyond with minimal or no pain complaints. Age, therefore, should not be a deterrent to walking. Pain during and after your walks may suggest that you are walking too hard, too fast, etc. Walking should not give you pain, and if it does, it should be a "pleasant" pain only.

Conclusion—Walk less, walk slower, hydrate, take breaks, include swimming and cycling in your training schedule and don't let age stop you! In fact, let age stimulate you!
—John Stanton

What causes stress fractures?

Bones, like a steel girder, under repetitive loading eventually fatigue and develop cracks. In the case of bones, this condition can be accelerated by inadequate support of the bones by the surrounding soft tissues, i.e., the muscles. These cracks lead to local pain and tenderness in the bone. Therefore, maintaining both ideal muscle strength and balance is the best way to avoid developing a stress fracture. Stress fractures occur most frequently in the shinbone (tibia), the foot (metatarsal) and the hip (femur or pelvis). Stress fractures occur in the foot bones in about 60% of cases and in the tibia or shinbone in 25%. Upper extremity injuries have also been reported but are extremely rare. Bones are the skeletal structures that provide anchors or attachments for the muscles, ligaments and tendons, so that they can exert force in order to generate movement. The bones also receive their strength from proper use of the adjacent muscles—so any situation where there is muscle weakness, anatomical conditions or misalignment can lead to weakening of the bones, which may lead to fractures. Maintaining bone health through proper nutrition is obvious. Adequate calcium and vitamin D are required. Beware of the female athlete triad—amenorrhea, anorexia and osteoporosis! This is a leading cause for the higher incidence of stress fractures in women.

The typical scenario of an athlete who is developing a stress fracture often begins with the non-diagnostic complaint of "my leg/foot/hip, etc., hurts after my long walk." Symptoms of a stress fracture can mimic those of shin splints, particularly early on in the condition. With continued walking the pain will progressively worsen. Initially, the pain improves with rest and avoidance of activity. However, until the fracture heals completely, the pain remains or may even get worse. Eventually, there is pain in the involved area with even simple movements such as walking slowly. If the affected bone is easily felt with your hand, there might be tenderness to touching it. There may be swelling in the area and the skin overlying the bone may seem warm. Eventually, especially if untreated, a stress fracture can lead to a complete break in the bone, thereby not even allowing you to stand without severe pain.

If you suspect you may have a stress fracture, the wisest thing to do is to curtail your walking for a week or two. Walking up until the point of pain is probably a practical suggestion for any injury. However, persistent pain is often the most important signal that something is amiss. The usual remedies of rest, ice and training modifications should always be tried first. Pain that does not go away, especially when there is also local bony tenderness, should alert the athlete to the possibility of an underlying stress fracture and you should visit your doctor.

—Dr. Richard Beauchamp

(For additional information on stress fractures please read Richard Beauchamp's articles on our website, www.runningroom.com.)

I want to train in the mountains; how does altitude affect my training?

As we increase the altitude above sea level the oxygen content of the air is reduced. The number of oxygen molecules is reduced and under resting conditions the individual can increase their rate of breathing to compensate for the limited amount of oxygen. The higher the altitude the more profound the effect. On a good note your maximal breathing capacity is greater at altitude than at sea level. There is also less air resistance at altitude. The air is also cooler and drier at a high altitude. This is good from a heat exchange standpoint but can also promote respiratory water loss. Another thing to consider is solar radiation is higher, so the use of sunscreen is even more important.

During the first few days at high altitude you may be less tolerant of lactate productions, but through a few days of adaptation and staying well hydrated you should notice little difference in your overall performance. If you are looking to compete in an event then my advice is to arrive a few days in advance and stick to your current training program. If you are fit and healthy to walk at sea then you will do equally well in altitude.

—John Stanton

What is a pedometer?

A pedometer is a device that clips to your belt or waistband and counts the number of steps you take. When your hip swings, an interior arm swings, too, causing a step to register on the display panel or counter.

I took a break from fitness walking over the winter. As I tried to get back into it this spring, I began getting a stitch in my right side, in the same place at the same time each walk. I've found that if I stop and stretch during this time, it works itself out but returns again. I've tried breathing differently, holding my arm above my head when I feel it coming on, massaging the area that hurts and nothing seems to be working. Any suggestions?

You are doing some of the things that will usually help alleviate what's commonly called "stitch." The truth of the matter is sports medicine professionals are not in agreement as to the cause of this discomfort.

One of the things I have found to work with walkers is to have them start off very slowly and gradually build up the intensity of their walk. Many have found that the sudden start to a walk and their labored breathing the first 10 minutes is the source of the discomfort.

Another thing to concentrate on is belly breathing. Concentrate on breathing deep in your diaphragm vs. high in your chest. Pursing your lips as you breathe out also helps in fully exhaling and relaxing the diaphragm. Try to really focus on staying as calm as possible and keep breathing relaxed and controlled.

All of us have a tendency to start walking with too much intensity, rather than with a gradual build-up of intensity.
—John Stanton

I am looking for a recommended way to breathe. I get a stitch. I have tried lots of stuff and found that exhaling all the air from the lungs seems to work. Should I try in from the nose out from the mouth or the other way around? Should I follow some sort of pattern?

Breathing, the simply act of inhaling and exhaling, can be complicated. Much like walking, the act of putting one foot in front of the other is a lot more complicated than one would expect. Watch the super talented singer who has mastered breathing. This mastery allows them to hit and hold the long high notes. Better yet, the swimmer has mastered breathing, if for no other reason than they do not want to get a mouth full of water. As walkers we occasionally get caught up in our sport and forget some basics like breathing. We start our walks in a race or group environment and the excitement causes us to breathe high in our chest rather than belly breathing. The short, high breathing can cause us to hyperventilate or get the dreaded stitch. Here are some tips that will make your stitch go away and get you more relaxed in your breathing, thereby, allowing you to walk faster.

Stand up tall, shoulders back and put one hand on your belly. Purse your lips and fully exhale. When we fully exhale we do not need to think about breathing in, as nature does this as part of our survival technique. We breathe in relaxed and belly breathe when we fully exhale. This deep breathing is both more relaxed and more efficient in the use of oxygen. Keep your breathing relaxed, deep, rhythmic and to time with your walking stride by concentrating on fully exhaling. Inhale in a relaxed, full, deep breath. So as you walk, concentrate on the upper body being relaxed and rhythmic, with the power of your walking focused on your hip down. The initial power is coming from the push off of the ankle

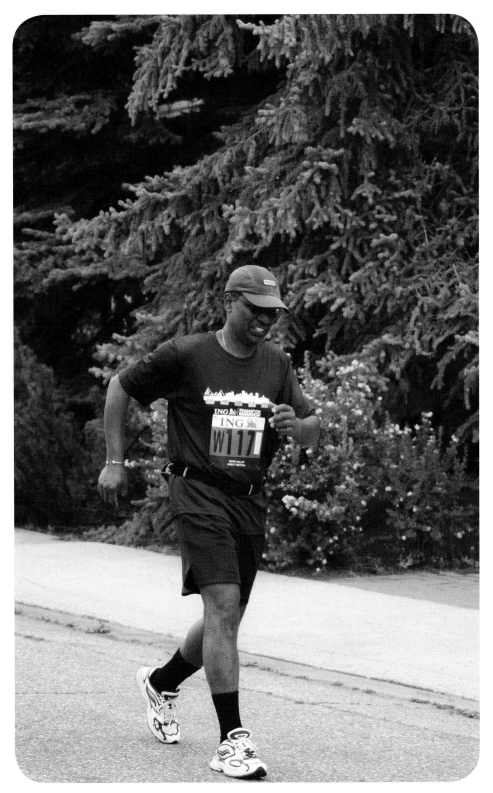

and the glide and relaxed lift of the knee coming from the hip flexors. Save the huffing and puffing for the big bad wolf stories. Now you know why one of the most common things a coach gets the athlete to concentrate on is to relax. The more relaxed we are the higher the level of performance. Enjoy your walking.
—John Stanton

Is walking on a treadmill the same as walking outdoors?

Treadmill walking is slightly easier than outdoor walking due to the lack of wind resistance. This enables you to be more efficient in your walking on the treadmill. To accommodate for the lack of resistance, increase the treadmill grade to about 2% for all of your workouts.

Walking on a treadmill is a great way to work on even pacing and to vary the intensity of your workouts. The intensity can be varied using a higher speed or a higher degree of incline for three to five minutes followed by three to five minutes of rest.

Long walks can be a social event with a non-walking buddy, or your latest TV show can take on a whole new perspective from the treadmill. Safety improves due to the controlled environment. As with your outdoor workouts, be sure to vary the intensity and duration of the workouts.
—John Stanton

How can I walk the marathon distance of 42 kilometers when the program training schedule longest walk is 32 kilometers?

Over the years, there have been a variety of training programs that overextend the long walk beyond the marathon distance. My experience is that the frequency of injury increases as we extend the long walk beyond the 32-km (20-mi) distance. I have seen too many folks walk a great long walk of 40–45 km. (25–28 mi) and then on marathon day come up with a disappointing time. The reason is that they did not give themselves enough time to recover from the long extended walk. Your training program is made up of base training, strength training and speed training. You train specifically in each phase; then on race day you put it all together and walk the marathon. Your distances should be looked at over a four-week period, not on one individual day. The taper phase of your training allows you to rest and recover from training and to perform to a higher standard on race day. Another key ingredient on race day is your adrenaline level, which, together with the group support and the crowd, will carry you the extra distance.

How can I walk my targeted pace in the marathon when I have walk my long training walks slower?

Slowing the long walks down helps you recover faster and gives you the desired endurance training effect while dramatically lowering your injury risk. You have plenty of hills, intervals and fartlek sessions to walk at race pace or faster to give you the speed. If you walked your long walks at nearly race pace, you would need more recovery. By slowing your pace by 15–20%, you will find that within a day or two you are ready to train hard, allowing you to do quality strength or speed work.

How can I prevent injury and be sure I take it to the start line?

Many talented walkers who approach their training in an overzealous manner end up sidelined by injury. Keep your training fun, keep it specific, keep it to the program and do not add to the program. Your training program is planned so that you will continually improve and get stronger. More is not necessarily better; fatigue will rob you of energy, both mentally and physically. Remember, walking is playtime!

How much of my total weekly distance should be speed?

Speed work should account for no more than 10–15% of your total weekly distance. Stick to the program and don't add any speed to your endurance training sessions. Training faster too often won't give your body enough time to recover between sessions.

We lose through water when walking. How much sodium and potassium do we lose? Can we take in too much water?

Recent media reports have made the issue of fluids and hydration very confusing, which is too bad, because if is actually a very straightforward issue. The American College of Sport Medicine (ACSM) says this about hydration, a statement that I completely endorse:

Hyponatremia is a dangerous condition that may arise when athletes consume too much water or sports drinks, diluting or disrupting the body's sodium levels. ACSM experts in sports medicine and exercise science point out that while hyponatremia is a serious concern, excessive fluid consumption resulting in hyponatremia is unlikely to occur in most athletes, and hydration is important for all active people. Water and sports drinks, when consumed as recommended, are not dangerous to athletes. And while hyponatremia has gotten more attention lately, far more athletes are affected by dehydration.

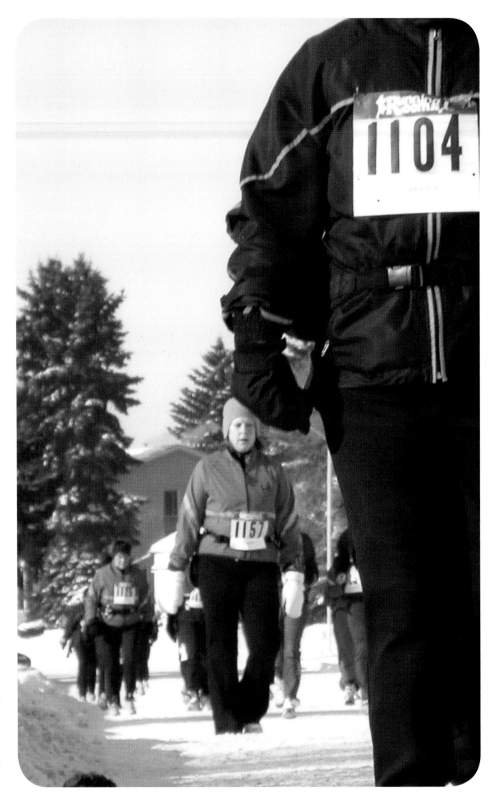

A good example of this comes from the experience at the 2004 Boston Marathon. According to *The Boston Globe*, "The main tent, which contained approximately 240 cots, was mostly full of dehydrated walkers complaining of nausea, diarrhea, and vomiting." Hospital officials reported a single case of hyponatremia in this year's marathon, involving a walker who was released after treatment."

With all of this in mind, it is truly unfortunate that the media and some individuals in the sport community have positioned over-hydration and hyponatremia as larger concerns than dehydration—the evidence paints quite a different picture if you really look at things.

The American College of Sport Medicine stands by its current advice on fluids and hydration:
- It is recommended that individuals drink about 500 ml (about 17 ounces) of fluid about two hours before exercise to promote adequate hydration and allow time for excretion of excess ingested water.
- During exercise, athletes should start drinking early and at regular intervals in an attempt to consume fluids at a rate sufficient to replace all the water lost through sweating (i.e., body weight loss), or consume the maximal amount that can be tolerated.
- It is recommended that ingested fluids be cooler than ambient temperature (between 15°C and 22°C, 59°F and 72°F).
- Fluids should be readily available and served in containers that allow adequate volumes to be ingested with ease and with minimal interruption of exercise.
- Addition of proper amounts of carbohydrates and/or electrolytes to a fluid replacement solution is recommended for exercise events of duration greater than one hour since it does not significantly impair water delivery to the body and may enhance performance. During exercise lasting less than one hour, there is little evidence of physiological or physical performance differences between consuming a carbohydrate-electrolyte drink and plain water.
- During intense exercise lasting longer than one hour, it is recommended that carbohydrates be ingested at a rate of 30–60 g/hour to maintain oxidation of carbohydrates and delay fatigue. This rate of carbohydrate intake can be achieved without compromising fluid delivery by drinking 600–1200 ml/hour of solutions containing 4–8% carbohydrates. (This the standard for most commercially produced sport drinks mixed to the manufacturers specifications.)
- Inclusion of sodium (0.5–0.7 g/liter of water) in the re-hydration solution

ingested during exercise lasting longer than one hour is recommended since it may be advantageous in enhancing palatability, promoting fluid retention, and possibly preventing hyponatremia in certain individuals who drink excessive quantities of fluid.

The full guidelines can be found at: www.acsm-msse.org/pt/pt-core/template-journal/msse/media/0196.htm. More information, based on the ACSM's "Position Stand on Exercise and Fluid Replacement," can be found on the Walking Room's website and in the electronic clinic manuals.

I hope this helps. I have certainly fielded a great number of questions about this recently. I hope this information clarifies things for our walkers.

Heidi M. Bates, BSc, RD
Nutrition Consultant
Tri-Nutrition Consulting

My wife walks about three times a week about 10K each walk. I'm sure she would walk more; however, she gets very nasty blisters on both of the feet, right on the instep. She has changed shoes three times, and yet the blisters continue. Is there something she can do?

The first thing to do is to pick up some liquid bandage or similar product. It is applied like a liquid. It will then dry and permit your wife to walk with some degree of comfort until the blisters heal. The next thing to do is to pick up a pair of Coolmax double layer socks to keep her feet cool and dry. The double layer works very well at preventing further blistering.

Change the lacing on the shoe to tighten up the heel area. Make two loops in the last lace holes at the top of her shoes and then bring the lace from the opposite side through the loop. Pull and tighten, then tie as normal. This will keep any heel slippage from occurring and hold her foot firmly in place.

Some Motivation Tips

+ Plan and schedule your daily workouts.
+ Be flexible within your schedule. Just commit to completing the workout.
+ Be creative in planning your workouts. Use normal downtime or waiting time to get in that walk, stretch session or cross-training session.
+ Read, listen to or watch something humorous. A good laugh gets rid of most stress.
+ Vary your workouts. Walking the same distance or course every day can

soon lead to boredom. A little speed or some hill repeats will put some spring back into your stride.

+ Walk with a buddy. You can motivate each other.
+ Imagine yourself in a race leading the pack that is 25 meters behind you. Push just a little.
+ In a safe area, put on headphones and listen to some music, a motivational clip or a comedy set.
+ Mix it up—change the time of day you normally walk; walk in a different direction; walk a new workout; or read a great new walking book.
+ Best yet, walk past a hospital to remind yourself how fortunate you are to have your good health. It is a fragile gift you must look after.
+ Savor each walk, as it is special in its own way.

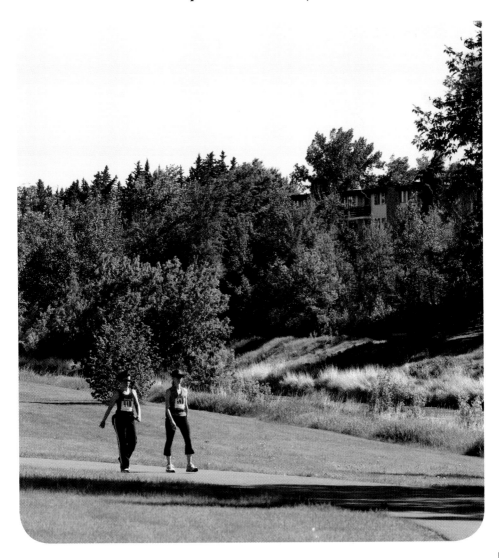

John Stanton
Founder of the Running Room

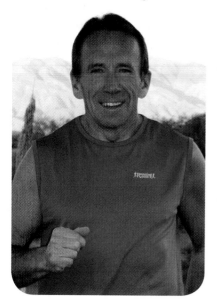

A best-selling Canadian author of four books on running and founder of the Running Room, John Stanton was named to *Maclean's* magazine's 2004 Canada Day Honor Roll as one of 10 Canadians making a difference in our nation for his contribution to health through fitness. John has also been featured on CBC Venture, the Vicki Gabereau show, Canada AM, CHUM Television, Global Television, the Weather Channel, the *National Post*, the *Globe and Mail*, and numerous radio and television programs across Canada and the United States.

A three-kilometer fun run with his young sons in 1981 was the catalyst that made then out-of-shape, overweight John Stanton realize he had to change his lifestyle. Then a food industry executive who smoked two packs of cigarettes a day, Stanton began running secretly before dawn because he felt self-conscious about having his neighbors see "this chubby little guy" who could only run from lamp post to lamp post before having to take a walk break.

In 1984 Stanton opened a store and meeting place for runners in an 8x10 foot room of an old house shared with a hairdressing shop in Edmonton, Alberta, Canada. Twenty years later, the Running Room he founded is one of North America's most recognized names in running and walking. In late 2004, to be more inclusive, his company launched the Walking Room—a mirror of the Running Room concept. The store caters specifically to the needs of walkers.

John Stanton has run more than 60 marathons, hundreds of road races and numerous triathlons, including the Canadian Ironman and the Ironman World Championship, Kona, Hawaii. His pre-dawn runs would ultimately become John Stanton's 10:1 run/walk combination that has helped well over 600,000 Canadians do everything from learn to run to complete marathons, upright and smiling.

Thousands of people have lost weight, improved their health and fitness levels and truly changed their lives as a result of one man who was determined to change his own life by losing weight and getting fit. John is now very active in working alongside cities such as Abbotsford, British Columbia, Edmonton, Alberta, Toronto, Ontario, and Moncton, New Brunswick, which have asked him and the Running Room to be part of community-wide fitness and weight awareness initiatives. John works with many charitable organizations and boards and is a vice president of the Commonwealth Games Association of Canada.

Biography

Acknowledgments

I would like to thank the great team of people who together provided their talents, infinite patience, skills and enthusiasm, as well as sharing in the vision of this book. This book, like most successful things in life, is about teamwork. To all friends, coaches, group leaders, clinic leaders, mentors, volunteers and family I say thank you.

Specifically I want to thank our Running Room team of Mike and Charlene O'Dell, Nancy Gillis for the design, layout and photography, Lee Craig for her meticulous proof reading and copy editing, Bev Stanton for her photography, John Reeves and Christina Leung for their product knowledge, Owen Archambault, Sue Henderson and Andy Wigston for their coaching feedback, and John, Jr., Jason and our families for the many hours spent on this project.

Special thanks to world walking experts Mark Fenton and Roger Burrows for their significant mentorship, encouragement, advice and ongoing efforts on spreading the word on walking.

I also would like to acknowledge the following individuals for their medical and technical advice: Harvey Sternberg, MD; Richard Beauchamp, MD; Julia Alleyne, BHSc(PT), MD; Jeffery Robinson, MD; Susan Glen, MSc, Nutrition; and Heidi Bates, BSc, RD.

Together let's celebrate the joy of walking.

John Stanton

Index of Select Terms

This index lists pages where you will find descriptions of various concepts and terms in the book. (It is not meant to be a comprehensive list for every time a word appears.)